the Unofficial Guide™ to Managing Eating Disorders

Sara Dulaney Gilbert with Mary C. Commerford, Ph.D.

IDG Books Worldwide, Inc.
An International Data Group Company
Foster City, CA • Chicago, IL • Indianapolis, IN
• New York, NY

W9-AYN-674

IDG Books Worldwide, Inc.
An International Data Group Company
919 E. Hillsdale Boulevard
Suite 400
Foster City, CA 94404

For general information on IDG Books Worldwide's books in the U.S., please call our Consumer Customer Service department at 800-762-2974. For reseller information, including discounts and previous sales, please call our Reseller Customer Service department at 800-434-3422.

ISBN: 0-02-862913-2

Manufactured in the United States of America

10 9 8 7 6 5 4 3 2 1

First edition

For Ian, in hindsight.
—Sara Dulaney Gilbert

Contents

The *Unofficial Guide* Reader's Bill of Rights

We give you more than the official line

Welcome to the *Unofficial Guide* series of Lifestyles titles—books that deliver critical, unbiased information that other books can't or won't reveal—*the inside scoop.* Our goal is to provide you with the *most accessible, useful* information and advice possible. The recommendations we offer in these pages are not influenced by the corporate line of any organization or industry; we give you the hard facts, whether those institutions like them or not. If something is ill-advised or will cause a loss of time and/or money, we'll give you ample warning. And if it is a worthwhile option, we'll let you know that, too.

Armed and ready

Our hand-picked authors confidently and critically report on a wide range of topics that matter to smart readers like you. Our authors are passionate about their subjects, but have distanced themselves enough from them to help you be armed and protected, and help you make educated decisions as you go through the process. It is our intent that, from having read this book, you will avoid the pitfalls everyone else falls into and get it right the first time.

Don't be fooled by cheap imitations; this is the genuine article *Unofficial Guide* series from IDG Books. You may be familiar with our proven track record of the travel *Unofficial Guides*, which have more than three million copies in print. Each year thousands of travelers—new and old— are armed with a brand new, fully updated edition of the flagship *Unofficial Guide to Walt Disney World*, by Bob Sehlinger. It is our intention here to provide you with the same level of objective authority that Mr. Sehlinger does in his brainchild.

The Unofficial panel of experts

Every work in the Lifestyle *Unofficial Guides* is intensively inspected by a team of two top professionals in their fields. These experts review the manuscript for factual accuracy, comprehensiveness, and an insider's determination as to whether the manuscript fulfills the credo in this Reader's Bill of rights. In other words, our Panel ensures that you are, in fact, getting "the inside scoop."

Our pledge

The authors, the editorial staff, and the Unofficial Panel of Experts assembled for *Unofficial Guides* are determined to lay out the most valuable alternatives available for our readers. This dictum means that our writers must be explicit, prescriptive, and above all, direct. We strive to be thorough and complete, but our goal is not necessarily to have the "most" or "all" of the information on a topic; this is not, after all, an encyclopedia. Our objective is to help you narrow down your options to the best of what is available, unbiased by affiliation with any industry or organization.

In each *Unofficial Guide* we give you:

- Comprehensive coverage of necessary and vital information

- Authoritative, rigidly fact-checked data

- The most up-to-date insights into trends

- Savvy, sophisticated writing that's also readable.

- Sensible, applicable facts and secrets that only an insider knows

Special features

Every book in our series offers the following six special sidebars in the margins that were devised to help you get things done cheaply, efficiently, and smartly.

1. **Timesaver**—tips and shortcuts that save you time

2. **Moneysaver**—tips and shortcuts that save you money

3. **Watch out!**—more serious cautions and warnings

4. **Bright Idea**—general tips and shortcuts to help you find and easier or smarter way to do something

5. **Quote**—statements from real people that are intended to be prescriptive and valuable to you

6. **Unofficially...**—an insider's fact or anecdote

We also recognize your need to have quick information at your fingertips, and have thus provided the following comprehensive sections at the back of the book:

1. **Glossary**—definitions of complicated terminology and jargon
2. **Resource Guide**—lists of relevant agencies, associations, institutions, Web sites, etc.
3. **Index**

Letters, comments, questions and from readers

We strive to continually improve the *Unofficial* series, and input from our readers is a valuable way for us to do that.

Many of those who have used the *Unofficial Guide* travel books write to the authors to ask questions, make comments, or share their own discoveries and lessons. For Lifestyle *Unofficial Guides*, we would also appreciate all such correspondence—both positive and critical—and we will make best efforts to incorporate appropriate readers' feedback and comments in revised editions of this work.

How to write to us:

Unofficial Guides
Lifestyle Guides
IDG Books
1633 Broadway
New York, NY 10019

Attention: Reader's Comments

About the Authors

Sara Dulaney Gilbert is the author of 25 self-help and useful-service books including, *Fat Free* and *You are What you Eat*. She has become a specialist in helping readers of all ages find their way through personal and physical changes and major life events. She has worked extensively in the field of higher education and holds a Master's degree from the Graduate School of Education at New York University. She resides in Cold Spring, New York.

Mary C. Commerford, Ph.D., a clinical psychologist, is the coordinator of the Eating Disorders Treatment Program at New York University. Prior to that, she was on the faculty at Cornell University Medical College, where she was involved with both treatment and research in eating disorders. She is the author of articles published in academic journals such as *The International Journal of Eating Disorders* and *Eating Disorders: Treatment and Prevention*. In addition, Dr. Commerford maintains a private practice in Manhattan.

The *Unofficial Guide* Panel of Experts

The *Unofficial* editorial team recognizes that you've purchased this book with the expectation of getting the most authoritative, carefully inspected information currently available. Toward that end, on each and every title in this series, we have selected a minimum of two "official" experts comprising the Unofficial Panel who painstakingly review the manuscripts to ensure the following: factual accuracy of all data; inclusion of the most up-to-date and relevant information; and that, from an insider's perspective, the authors have armed you with all the necessary facts you need—but that the institutions don't want you to know.

For *The Unofficial Guide to Managing Eating Disorders,* we are proud to introduce the following panel of experts:

Sibyl M. Wagner, M.S.W., C.C.S.W., received her A.B. in Psychology from the University of North Carolina at Chapel Hill in 1973. In 1975 she graduated from the School of Social Work at the University of Pennsylvania. She first worked as a Clinical Social Worker at the teaching hospitals for the University of North Carolina and then for the University of California, San Diego. She has been in private practice since January 1980, with a special interest in eating disorders. In addition, she has served as a Clinical Assistant Professor in the U.N.C. School of Medicine, Dept. of Psychiatry from 1984–1998. She has been active in bringing the dangers of eating disorders to the public (especially young people) through a variety of media, including television and radio,as well as workshops and other educational presentations.

Lisa Mandelbaum, MS, RD, CD-N, received her Master of Science degree in Clinical Nutrition from Hunter College, School of Health Sciences. She maintains a full-time private nutrition practice on the Upper West Side of Manhattan in New York City. A Registered Dietitian, she provides counseling to individuals with a variety of nutritional concerns including eating disorders, weight management, pregnancy and lactation, sports nutrition, gastrointestinal disorders, and overall wellness. Recently, she was a nutrition specialist and coordinator of patient care and counseling at Peak Wellness in Greenwich, Connecticut, where she provided nutritional counseling and led community outreach programs at local public and private schools.

Introduction

An estimated 8 million people in the United States, and countless others around the world, suffer from eating disorders—anorexia nervosa, bulimia, and binge eating, among them. For this reason alone, this book's information and advice on managing eating disorders from both professionals and survivors is important.

The fact that eating disorders have received so much attention in recent years is a healthy sign, even if there has been a fair amount of media hype, in some cases. But eating disorders are not new or fad diseases—nor do they affect only affluent young women, despite what some media coverage might suggest. Eating disorders are potentially fatal maladies that afflict a wide variety of people from an equally wide range of backgrounds. They stem from complex social, psychological, physical, and emotional roots.

Whether you suspect an eating disorder in yourself or in someone close to you—or if you simply want to understand what's behind some of today's hyped-up headlines—this book will give you an inside look at the facts. It also will help you gain firsthand insights into the compulsions that drive these devastating conditions. Here you'll find the results of the latest research on anorexia nervosa, bulimia, Binge eating disorder, and other syndromes, as well as a thorough exploration of the most effective treatments.

This book also guides you through the complexities of these often baffling disorders and offers suggestions for workable solutions. The good news is, despite all the headlines and photos that may scare you about these disorders, they *are* treatable, and you can take steps to help a loved one. *But*, treatment and action are necessary, as we'll explain.

Why this book is important now

Eating disorders have come out of the closet. The fact that so many celebrities are going public about their compulsions means that more ordinary citizens may feel more comfortable about both acknowledging and seeking treatment for eating disorders. The fact that awareness has increased may not make the problem any easier to solve, but it does make it seem less shameful. Taking the first step toward treatment is easier when you have a more realistic understanding of the sources and extent of an eating disorder. Therefore, Part I, "Food, Body Image, and Self-Esteem," offers a clear-headed, commonsense view of how and why eating disorders develop.

The new openness about eating disorders shows that they are more pervasive than once thought, especially when you take into account all the people who don't completely fit the extreme stereotypical profiles of anorexia or bulimia but who suffer from an eating disorder nonetheless.

In fact, with each discovery researchers make about eating disorders, the more we realize how complex and dangerous these conditions are. The greater our understanding of the facts, the better the chances of successfully managing these disorders. Part II, "Eating Disorders," provides the very latest information about anorexia, bulimia, Binge Eating Disorder, and a host of others. Each chapter includes definitions, warning signs, and symptoms, as well as moving and powerful testimonials from people who have experienced and survived these devastating disorders.

Dangerous disorders

There's no question that eating disorders *are* dangerous: They can do great damage to the body in a variety of ways and can even be fatal if they are left untreated. People who use drugs to stimulate vomiting, bowel movement, or urination are in the most danger because these practices increase the risk of heart failure. In patients who have anorexia, starvation can damage vital organs such as the heart and kidneys and can cause shrinkage of the brain. These conditions can be reversed, however, with treatment. Still, most experts consider "curing" eating disorders difficult, mainly because eating disorders are prone to relapse. Early detection and treatment lead to a better prognosis and faster remission of symptoms, which make these potentially chronic illnesses that much easier to live with and manage.

Socially destructive conditions

Eating disorders may be reaching epidemic proportions in the United States, where as many as 20 percent of some age groups (especially adolescents and young adults) are stricken with symptoms ranging from mildly disordered eating patterns to full-fledged anorexia and bulimia. Although it can be argued that enhanced reporting of these diseases is responsible for a heightened national awareness of them, it is also an indication of how pervasive they really are.

But the universality of eating disorders is not their worst aspect: Age of onset is earlier than ever before, meaning that these conditions are affecting children who are as young as 8 years old. Whenever children are affected by something as insidious as eating disorders, society's alarm bells should ring especially loud. Still, it is particularly difficult to admit that a child is well into a destructive pattern of behavior or has a serious health condition.

The sooner the symptoms are recognized, however, the greater the hope for recovery. That's why Part III, "Responding to Danger Signals," shares professional and first-person advice on how to detect an eating disorder and what to do if you uncover one. (The rule of thumb is this: If you suspect an eating disorder in someone you know—or even in yourself— chances are good that there is one.) Here you'll find valuable information about techniques that work—and those that don't.

In Part IV, "Treatments for Eating Disorders," we summarize the treatments, from cognitive behavior and insight therapies to 12-step programs, group therapy, and support groups. We discuss denial, fear, and other difficult roadblocks to recovery; and we share the joys, disappointments, surprises, and revelations of getting better. Here, too, are the voices and testimony of real people who have lived through the disorders and survived them. We offer the best information we could find on how to evaluate and cover the costs of treatment, and which networks you should trust for reliable information and support.

Treatable conditions

It sounds absurdly simple: If you have a problem, get help for it. But if it were that easy, no one would suffer for years or die from an eating disorder. As we discover more about these subtle, deeply rooted disorders, the variety of treatments increases and become more successful at attacking them from every angle, through a combination of psychological, medical, nutritional, and pharmacological approaches.

Given the enhanced awareness of and increased success in treating eating disorders, the need for up-to-the-minute information is especially critical. That's what this book provides. At the same time, we go beyond facts and information, and provide practical guidance about treatment—how to enhance recovery and prevent a relapse, for example—which you will find not only in Part IV, but throughout the book.

Scientists who are actively studying ways to treat and understand eating disorders are engaged in complex explorations of biochemical interactions. But their research continues to confirm the simple fact that people who get early treatment for eating disorders have a better chance of full recovery than those who wait years before getting help. Nevertheless, it can be quite difficult to get people into treatment, an eventuality the book addresses with both practical tips and more scientific information.

The family factor

It is also true that for every incidence of the disease, a family is torn apart and every person who is stricken faces potential damage for a lifetime, even after specific symptoms are relieved. Part V, "Living with Someone Who Has an Eating Disorder," focuses especially on the challenges of living with a loved one with this type of disorder—and getting help for that, too.

In addition to the seriousness and complexity of eating disorders, denial is a key characteristic. Sometimes this means that people in the grips of an eating disorder may not realize it. In many cases, they defy anyone who raises the subject with them and resist all efforts of treatment. Even the families of people whose eating is quite clearly disordered often refuse to acknowledge the problem. In truth, they may not be able to see what is obvious to everyone else. This is why reaching people who need treatment or even information can be difficult.

Throughout the book, we provide stories and information that will strike a familiar chord for anyone who has been touched by an eating disorder. We urge you to respond to that sense of connection by taking steps toward getting help, whether for yourself or for a loved one. As the last sections of the book point out, a positive approach to an eating disorder usually leads to a positive outcome.

How to make best use of this book

This book makes the most reliable facts accessible so that people who *need* the facts can find them *easily*. It also offers firsthand insights into what the diseases are really like, to encourage and hopefully make it easier for people to reach out for help. Whether you approach the book from cover to cover, go to the topics that concern you the most, or simply browse to get a sense of what you need to know, we've tried to make it easy to get information and gain understanding of eating disorders.

The latest facts

For this book we have gathered information from a wide range of research in the fields of medicine, psychology, and social science to provide detailed information that delineates eating disorders and the various means of treating them.

The profile of what once was considered the "typical" person who has anorexia or bulimia may surprise you. And did you know that an entirely new class of eating disorder has recently been defined? Or that new biochemical research has yielded promising new treatment possibilities?

We acknowledge that even the most comprehensive collection of facts may not be complete and that not everyone will be able to find certain information that applies specifically to his individual case. That's why we've provided a thorough listing of the associations and organizations that deal with every aspect of eating disorders—groups for sufferers, professional societies, medical researchers, and online access. We've also included lists of books and other valuable publications on the subject.

An effective format

The facts alone can help define a disorder, even for people who are in denial or who are indirectly affected by an eating disorder. Therefore the facts are presented here as often as possible in lists, sidebars, and other formats that help make the reality of a disorder clearly apparent. Experts know that the more facts a person encounters about her situation, the less able she will be to deny the truth.

True stories

One of the most powerful tools for recovery from eating disorders is the experience of other people.

No matter how sophisticated the psychological research or how advanced the pharmacological applications, one of the most effective means of reaching people with eating disorders is hearing the stories of people like themselves. Their accounts vividly demonstrate the reality of often bizarre-sounding facts and underscore the key facts about eating disorders. These disorders are progressive and can result in death if not treated; even when a disorder is only limited or chronic, it can make life more difficult and painful than it need be.

Throughout this book, we've included the personal experiences of people who have been challenged by eating disorders of all kinds. Note that in all cases, the identities of the people whose stories are shared here are altered or paraphrased to protect their privacy. Still, anyone who can identify with the stories of others whose problems are similar to her own is on the way to finding a solution.

How to make the best use of this information

Because eating disorders are so complex, and because the emotions that drive them are so powerful, one of the most effective antidotes is simply to get the facts. If you can absorb and apply the facts to the condition that concerns you, a friend, or a member of your family, they may be all that you need. Facts aren't a magic bullet, of course, but they can go a long way toward demystifying difficult information, clarifying objectives, and making it that much less daunting to plan treatment and recovery for yourself or someone you know.

If you can make contact with one of the many organizations devoted to eating-disorder research and recovery, you've taken a step in a positive direction. In fact, if all this guide does is point you or someone you know to a group that can provide help, it will have accomplished an important end.

Simply passing the book along to someone with an eating disorder can provide help as well. People who have eating disorders are usually extremely isolated; they feel they are alone in their situation. Hopefully this book will help break their isolation and give them the courage to seek help.

If your suspicions about another person's disorder are strengthened by reading any of the material here, then the best thing you can do is take some sort of action. Eating disorders pose a serious threat to health and even have the potential to kill. Use your newly acquired knowledge to help someone else grasp that reality—it could save a life.

You have taken the first step toward helping yourself or someone you know just by picking up this book. We hope that the expert information, advice, and personal experiences in these pages will carry you the rest of the way.

Food, Body Image, and Self-Esteem

PART I

GET THE SCOOP ON...
Twisted self-images ▪ Irresistible compulsions ▪
The need for emotional nourishment ▪ The
power of the family ▪ Social stresses

The Causes of Eating Disorders

Chapter 1

Anyone who's ever been close to someone who has an eating disorder has likely wondered in despair, "Why can't she just stop?" or, "Can't he see what he's doing to himself?" That, of course, is the point: People who have eating disorders *can't* stop. They can't "see" clearly.

Anorexia, bulimia, and other food-related compulsions do not stem from willful behavior or bad habits, but from serious, deep-rooted, physical and emotional disorders. These disorders are devastating in their effects on the physical, emotional, and social aspects of a person's life—and their causes are complex.

Although not all experts agree exactly on the source of specific motivators for eating disorders, most specialists point to a similar set of causes. According to the Surgeon General of the United States, "Most theories about the sources—or causal factors—of eating disorders fall into four categories:

Unofficially...
The American
Anorexia/Bulimia
Association
(AABA) notes
that scientists
have studied the
personalities,
genetics, envi-
ronments, and
biochemistry of
people with
these illnesses.
As is often the
case, the more
that is learned,
the more com-
plex the roots of
eating disorders
appear.

organic, psychodynamic, familial, and sociocul-
tural." In other words, look for the sources of these
destructive behaviors in the body, the mind, the family, society—and in all the links between them.

Keep in mind, though, that while this chapter
details the causal factors of eating disorders as they
are identified by experts, what really drives people
to these essentially self-destructive behaviors is a
powerful inner force that can best be explained by
those who have experienced it. Their words, in this
chapter and elsewhere in the book, are as important
as any scientific explanation of these devastating disorders.

Body image: A reflection of inner feelings

What people do to themselves when they use food as
a weapon is closely tied to how they see themselves
physically and how they feel about themselves
emotionally.

People who have disordered eating patterns also
have disordered perceptions: They see themselves as
"fat" and, by their definitions, "not good enough"
because in the American culture, being thin is
equated with being good. As these people see it, if
they are fat, they are not really good enough inside.
They feel that they can't fix this internal reality, so
they focus on changing the external one: their
appearance.

Bright Idea
To gain a deeper
understanding of
the complex
inner forces
behind eating
disorders, attend
an open meeting
of a support or
recovery group
for people strug-
gling with
anorexia and
bulimia, and lis-
ten to their
experiences first-
hand.

This process of externalizing an interior conflict—the perception that one is too fat—is not
conscious or rational, and it's usually not based on
reality, either. But for people who have an eating
disorder, self-perception is very real. Even if what
they see—an image of themselves as "fat"—is *not*
real, what is being projected from within—a deep-
set negative feeling about themselves—*is* real.

The American Anorexia/Bulimia Association has learned from its members that the compulsions serve as "an expression of what the person has found no other way of expressing—typically feelings of shame, doubt, rage, grief, inadequacy." Furthermore, they perceive that they are not being recognized as separate beings; that they are "unseen, unknown, and unaccepted for who they are."

Eating disorders often emerge in early puberty, a time when some girls naturally gain weight to support the initiation of hormonal cycles. This makes them especially vulnerable to critical messages from those around them—particularly about being "pudgy." Eating disorders are almost tailor-made for girls at this transitional stage of life. Another risky time occurs when students go away to college. Leaving home, family, and friends to face new social challenges can be tremendously stressful, especially when other students with whom they come into contact and who already have eating disorders inadvertently set an example for the uninitiated. Anxiety; stress; and competition about grades, excelling, and making the team, also provide a rich breeding ground for all kinds of disordered eating.

Narrowing the profile

Teens tend to be edgy and self-conscious, of course, but not all of them develop food disorders. What makes the difference? Specialists note that people who develop these disorders tend to be overly sensitive and attuned to others, especially as youngsters. The theory is that their acute sensitivity to the needs of other people teaches them to avoid acting on anger so as not to upset others. As these youths grow older, they suppress difficult feelings deeper and deeper within themselves. As preteens and

When I was a teenager, I was interested in boys but didn't think I was pretty enough to get their attention. Once my father said, I guess as a joke, that I would never get a date if I didn't take off some weight. I took him very him seriously and began to diet until I couldn't stop.
—A young woman, now recovering from anorexia nervosa

teenagers, they often are considered "too good to be true" by friends, teachers, family, and schoolmates. Indeed, they are rarely disobedient, excel whenever they are expected to do so, and tend to be perfectionists.

However, these outward characteristics very often mask inner turmoil and feelings of self-loathing. At the same time, teenagers whose *outward* behavior is negative, rebellious, and out of control may turn to pathological dieting with the same zeal as peers whose inner conflicts are less visible.

Some researchers believe that people who have anorexia focus on food restrictions (eating too little) as a means to gain a sense of control in at least one area of their lives, which helps explain why so many teenagers suffer from this disorder. Even some adults who have always followed the wishes of others may not have learned how to cope on their own with issues related to adolescence, growing up, and becoming independent. For them, controlling their weight appears to have a double benefit, at least at first: They can take control of their bodies and also gain approval from others.

Feelings of inadequacy are common to most of us, of course. Surveys show that more than half of American women think (erroneously) that they are too fat. Yet only a small percentage of them react by trying to control their food in a disordered or pathological fashion.

Overwhelming drives

Eating disorders involve obsessive-compulsive behaviors. That is, sufferers experience a *compulsion*—an irresistible inner force—to commit an irrational act, and they are fueled by an *obsession*—a persistent, unshakable idea that is rooted in an unhealthy mental or emotional state.

The fact that eating disorders are the products of obsessions and compulsions, and that they are profoundly self-destructive, as well, indicates to many psychologists that eating disorders are indeed eloquent expressions of deep underlying problems.

A crazy kind of sense

Most people who have eating disorders are extremely sensitive and have trouble expressing their emotions. In anorexia, bulimia, and Binge Eating Disorder, eating behaviors often seem to develop as a way of handling stress, anxiety, and difficult emotions. Indeed, hunger and purging *can* numb painful emotions, while compulsive behaviors provide distraction from deeper disturbances.

Someone who has created the need to focus a great deal of energy and attention on regulating food, weight, and exercise doesn't really have the time to pay attention to painful issues and events in life, such as struggling for good grades, or facing a divorce.

The compulsive process itself is about control. Compulsive behaviors provide predictability and comfort when life feels out of control and chaotic. People who are obsessive-compulsive about eating have rigid rituals around food: They may eliminate certain foods from their diet, for example, or develop patterns, such as cutting food into very small pieces. This behavior tends to be progressive; as the individual becomes more obsessive, the ability to manage feelings and personal relationships gets lost, resulting in emotional emptiness and withdrawal. Compulsive behavior is an attempt to control both one's self and one's relationships with others.

People who develop bulimia and Binge Eating Disorder typically consume huge amounts of

Unofficially...
Though self-starvation must be addressed, most experts agree that food and eating habits are *not* the central problem of MOST eating disorders. Rather, food is used as a tool for coping. With food people gain an increased sense of control and self-esteem, and this helps them manage difficult emotions, such as anger, albeit in an indirect way.

Watch Out!
The AABA warns that an eating disorder is not only a problem but also an attempted *solution* to a problem, so underlying causes present considerable dangers.

66

I was finally able to admit that I had a problem with food and began to understand that my obsession with food was only the symptom of deeper, underlying emotional issues when I learned to use a few tools that helped me deal with my feelings instead of using food as a means to numb out.
—A woman in her 30s who has had anorexia for twenty years

99

food—often junk food—to reduce stress and relieve anxiety. But instead of bringing relief, excessive eating brings guilt and depression. Purging can provide relief, but it is only temporary. By restricting food, bingeing, or bingeing and purging, that person can shift the focus to something other than the struggle to cope with family members, significant others, or a major change, such as going to college.

Thus, the food-related problems that seem insane at first, aren't so crazy after all. In some ways, they are a very effective way of dealing with great pain. When food disorders are seen as efforts to control life's problems, they actually make a crazy kind of sense.

Pathological patterns

The problem is, of course, that this crazy kind of sense is based on distorted perceptions and an inability to see reality. Certain behaviors that may appear to be self-destructive to an observer are, to the person who has an eating disorder, the logical outcome of his thinking.

In particular, some people who have anorexia nervosa exhibit "all-or-nothing" thinking: They see everything in black-and-white categories. For example, an A– is considered a "bad grade." When it comes to food, there are only two choices: to starve or to be fat. There is no middle ground. If any effort is not "perfect," then it is a total failure. People who have anorexia tend to filter out any information that doesn't fit into their scheme. They see only the negative and dwell on it as if it were an all-pervasive pattern.

Without regarding the facts, some people who have eating disorders conclude that everything they do is negative and will have negative results. They distort facts by exaggerating or denigrating them, and then they use emotional reasoning to prove that the situation is really the way they see it. A college student confronting difficult challenges on her own for the first time may come to feel that if she were "good enough," she could handle all her challenges successfully. "Good enough" comes to mean "slender," so she starts a rigid diet. Failing at that, she turns to her emotional reasoning, which tells her that this failure "proves" that she's no good. Her response is to diet even more strictly, and the cycle worsens.

Another irrational pattern that characterizes the thinking of people with eating disorders is the repeating of the same behavior and expecting different results. Life becomes so painful that they seek food to alleviate the discomfort, even though this has never worked in the past. According to Dr. Christopher Fairburn (of Oxford University, England), who developed a model for bulimia, the pattern follows this progression:

Low self-esteem leads to extreme concerns with body shape and weight, which leads to strict dieting. Dieting causes more anxiety, which triggers binge eating and purging. Bad feelings about the binge/purge cycle cause a repeat in the process, which, of course, leads to even lower self-esteem and keeps the cycle in process.

Hungry for what?

Psychologists explain that everyone needs emotional nourishment, beginning in early infancy—when cuddling and snuggling are almost as important as food—and extending through youth and into adulthood.

It is easy to see how food—and the physical and emotional contact that come with it—is so important to an infant. A baby's first important activity

Timesaver
There's little point in trying to reason with someone who has anorexia, bulimia, or any other food compulsion. These people are simply unable to respond positively to rational arguments.

Moneysaver
To get more information about other aspects of eating disorders without paying a fortune, get in touch with the associations that sponsor support and research. Or, go to their sites on the World Wide Web. You'll get the latest, unbiased information, for free. Check out Appendix B, "Resource Guide," for a list of reputable sites.

outside her mother's body is eating. Her first contact with the world is through her mouth. And, of course, eating is vitally important to growth and well-being. Although a baby's cry may say simply, "I'm hungry," the hunger that is satisfied by a feeding is not just for food. When most young babies are fed, they are also held snugly and comfortably. Is it any surprise that adults turn to food when they need comfort, too?

There's nothing pathological about indulging in a favorite "comfort food" after a tough day. However, problems *do* arise when food is used as one's sole coping strategy, or when food becomes the single focus of one's search for emotional nourishment. The need to be loved, accepted, supported, and encouraged doesn't disappear with babyhood. Children seek these supports from their families and then from their friends; teenagers and adults turn to peers, work, and romantic attachments.

No relationship—whether with family, friends, or lovers—can be the perfect, most complete source of all emotional nourishment. But when some people feel let down by a relationship, they react by turning their anger and disappointment with the other person or the situation against themselves. They believe very intensely that something is wrong with *them*.

Why do some people turn on themselves in this way? The reasons aren't yet clear, but experts feel that one likely source is within the family.

The power of the family

A recent study found that mothers who are overly concerned about their daughters' weight and physical attractiveness inadvertently put the girls at an increased risk of developing eating disorders. Girls

"
While I was visiting a patient who had been hospitalized for anorexia, I couldn't help overhearing what her mother said: 'Dear, why *don't* you put on a little makeup? You want to look nice, don't you?' —A psychologist who specializes in treating people who have anorexia
"

whose fathers and brothers are overly critical of their weight are susceptible as well.

Families are far from being the only cause of eating disorders, but sometimes they *do* create environments that foster them. For example, some people who have anorexia claim that excessive dieting has given them a greater sense of control over their lives and more independence from overprotective or overly rigid parents.

Specialists who study the families of people who have eating disorders find that they are "too enmeshed." In other words, families in which the relationships are too closely tied together tend not to have emotional boundaries, which makes it difficult for children to create their own identities. The message these families send to their children is that the world is a dangerous place that can't be negotiated safely. This attitude necessitates the development of rigid, compulsive systems for coping with the outside world. Or, a family may be the opposite—so uncaring that they force children out on their own, emotionally. But what is it about food that makes it such a powerfully protective weapon?

Family messages and self-esteem

In some families food is presented in the spirit of parental acceptance and support, and as a means of providing children with the energy to pursue their own lives. It is unlikely that an eating disorder would develop in the context of this family.

On the other hand, some parents serve food to their children along with the message that they consider good looks and especially slenderness a sign of success. Therefore, food is withheld or controlled as a disciplinary measure in the pursuit of slim bodies. In some families, food is clearly offered as a form of

Watch Out!
Parents create food problems without even knowing it: "Oh, you're such a good baby to finish your cereal." "Behave and I'll give you a lollipop." When food is used as a punishment or a reward, it takes on power far beyond its value as nutrition.

love, and children who do not eat it are seen to be rejecting their parents. In these situations, children may learn to eat—or not eat—as a weapon to protect themselves from an overwhelming parental presence.

Just as one family pattern is to overwhelm children with too much food and love, another may convey the message that whatever a child does, it is never good enough. Parents may mean well by this—they may only want to urge their children to "be better." But a sensitive child who is already predisposed to disordered eating may respond by using food to strive for perfection.

Socially acceptable disorders

Can we blame eating disorders all on the family? Of course not. Still, our culture insists that all of us—women, in particular—should be slender, or at least should spend a lot of time and energy trying to become thinner. Swallowing cultural messages about the value of slenderness leads many people—again, girls and women, in particular—to mistrust their bodies and brains. They feel tremendous pressures to diet to be slim and have a "fat-free" body.

In the long run, men and women who diet below the set point—the ideal weight the body has chosen—can fall into cycles of binge eating and promote weight gain. (See Chapter 16, "In Balance," for more details about set point.) People who buy into this diet game run the risk of developing an eating disorder.

Each person's body weight and shape, like his or her intelligence and personality, is unique. Like it or not, our genes are the primary influence in establishing a specific weight range for each of us. Some people are simply destined to be heavier or lighter than others.

In the American culture, however, we simply don't believe that. Dieting is an integral part of many people's lives. In recent years, exercise has also become a vital part of this culture. And just as dieting is an acceptable way for teens to act out, focusing our energies on exercise has become a socially acceptable way for adults to cope with the stresses of life.

Exercise is good for you, right? Low-fat eating is healthy, right? Certainly this is true, but as in so many other areas, it's possible to carry a good thing too far.

The dieting dilemma

Under the influence of powerful cultural forces, many people believe that body weight is a personal statement, without ever stopping to question their logic. Because they equate body weight with the number of calories that go in and go out, they assume that people can control how much they weigh. In a culture that considers being slender and firm as the ultimate good, most of us are pressured to diet or do whatever it takes to become slender and get rid of body fat.

The irrational interior dialogue goes like this: If the process of restricting and controlling food makes you hungry, or if you feel preoccupied and irritable, it's just a sign that you lack self-control and must apply yourself all the more to the important task of weight management.

Though you wouldn't know it from the magazine headlines at the supermarket checkout, scientific research has a completely different take on weight and dieting. Most people's daily intake of

Unofficially...
Although most people who suffer from anorexia and bulimia are adolescent and young adult women, these illnesses also strike men and older women. Anorexia and bulimia are found most often in Caucasians, but these illnesses also increasingly affect Asian Americans and African Americans. People who pursue professions or activities that emphasize thinness—such as modeling, dancing, gymnastics, wrestling, and long-distance running—are more susceptible to the problem.

Unofficially...
Case studies of people who have developed eating disorders such as anorexia nervosa and bulimia reveal that more than 80 percent of the cases began with dieting.

66

My struggle started with a normal diet during my last year of high school. When I saw how the weight dropped off, I kept on pushing myself to lose 'just' 10 more pounds to make sure I would stay skinny. After being treated for anorexia, I resorted to bingeing and purging, which was a living hell. I isolated myself from everyone and was angry all of the time. Honestly, I never thought I would get over it.
—A college student, now recovered

99

food and expenditure of energy vary a great deal over the course of two or three months, yet their average body weight varies only slightly. Careful studies of weight-loss programs demonstrate over and over again that people *can* lose weight—even a lot of weight—in the short run. But, perhaps because of the body's drive to return to its set point, less than 5 percent will keep the weight off. In fact, many will regain all the weight they lost, if not more.

Peer pressure

The vast majority—more than 90 percent—of those afflicted with eating disorders are adolescent and young adult women. Approximately 1 percent of adolescent girls develop anorexia nervosa; another 2 to 3 percent of young women develop bulimia. In large part, this is because these groups in particular are vulnerable to peer pressures to be slender. The idea of being different is horrifying to these people; because they are all bathed in the same media images that glamorize slim bodies, none of them wants to be "fat." Feeling pressured to be thin, they go on diets that evolve into serious eating disorders, in some cases.

In women's dorms and dining halls on college campuses, not eating is reported to be a way of life: These young women take pride in how little they've consumed in a given day. Consequently, eating-disorder centers are becoming as commonplace on campuses across the country as career centers.

Screening images

The media—movies, advertisements, television shows, and so on—fill our minds and flood our senses with very slim bodies that match only 3 percent of the American population, experts say. Yet these are the ideal body shapes we are expected to strive for. Conflicts regarding food are plain to see on the TV screen: There are almost as many ads for snacks and beer as there are for diet programs and exercise machines. No wonder young people are so confused!

At the same time that our culture teaches us to value people for themselves, our media reflects the reality that people are valued for their bodies more than anything else. This applies to women and girls, especially, even in this "politically correct" era. But it applies to men, too: *Baywatch,* the world's most watched TV program, has as many "beautiful" male bodies as female ones.

It is also due to the "slim-is-good" school of thought that many people live with eating disorders without realizing it. Surprisingly, some eating-disorder specialists define the ideal weight as "one that can be maintained comfortably, while eating a full range of foods, without restrictions." Even more surprising to hear is their suggestion that we throw away our scales!

So what's the result of so many mixed messages? Take a culture that bombards us with messages about the importance of beautiful, slim bodies; feed it to people who have a certain biochemical makeup (and who have received the message from family and friends that they are not "good enough"); and you have all the social, psychological, and physiological ingredients for the development of a full-fledged eating disorder.

Then, because it is so acceptable now to be very slim, it can take a long time to recognize that someone close to us is getting entirely *too* thin. And if it takes too long for *us* to recognize this condition, it can be too late for *that person* because some eating disorders are fatal.

Watch Out!
One of the most frightening aspects of anorexia nervosa is that people who have the disorder continue to think that they are over-weight, even when they are bone thin.

Just the facts

- Anorexia, bulimia, bingeing, and other eating disorders are the products of a combination of psychological, physiological, familial, and social factors.

- Eating disorders are physical compulsions driven by mental obsessions.

- Eating disorders serve as powerful tools in an individual's struggle for self-expression.

- Eating disorders can easily be masked as "socially acceptable" behavior.

- Understanding the causes of eating disorders is critical, but often the causes are subtle, under the surface, and not immediately clear to either the sufferer or his family and friends.

GET THE SCOOP ON...
The power of media messages ▪ Weight-myths
and realities ▪ Distorted body images ▪ When
the weight-game kicks off ▪ Self-image and eating disorders

Body Image

W ith Barbie dolls and GI Joes, children
are given an early introduction to body
image and the shapes and sizes that are
most desirable in our culture. These plastic dolls
show children the way people "are supposed" to
look, just as the near-naked bodies on *Baywatch,* one
of the most popular TV shows in the world, remind
young adults (and older ones, too) what perfect
bodies should look like.

Whatever the specific causes, most experts agree
that disordered perceptions of the body contribute
to eating disorders. Misperceptions of the body
would probably occur even without media portrayals,
but the fact that images of the "ideal body" permeate
the culture has a lot to do with setting unattainable
physical standards.

It would be hard to find anyone in modern
America who thought she had a perfect body or who
didn't compare herself unfavorably with models or
actors. But for the vulnerable, a distorted body
image is a key factor in triggering eating disorders.

Chapter 2

Who says you're too fat or too thin?

In cultures where food is scarce, fatness is a sign of prosperity, leisure, and wealth. In the United States, however, where food is abundant, the sign of prosperity and leisure is being very thin.

Researchers note that women depicted in magazines have been getting thinner over the past two decades. During the height of the "fit is in" period, "fit" meant bony in women's magazines. This was followed by a spate of "heroin chic" advertisements featuring models whose gauntness looked almost horrifying.

The average model in women's clothing ads and the average mannequin in most stores is tall, weighs 120 pounds, and wears a size 6, at a time when the average American woman is 5 feet, 4 inches, weighs about 140 pounds, and wears a size 12. A similar discrepancy exists between male clothing models and actual male bodies.

Although the fashion industry continues to model small sizes, clothing manufacturers are producing an increasing number of large sizes to accommodate the size of real women.

Who's too thin and who's too fat? It would seem that the models are "too thin," but the public thinks of itself as "too fat." Some experts have voiced their amazement that *all* American women don't have anorexia, given the pressures of the market. Young women who desperately want to fit in, and who have the least experience in separating image from reality, are the ones most affected by media messages about weight.

The irony, of course, is that the glowing images projected by the media as the end products of serious dieting very often result in dry, lackluster skin

> 66
> This exercise system is fabulous! I've dropped from a size 7 to a size 4—and now my clothes just hang off of me!
> —A young woman promoting an exercise video on TV
> 99

and hair, as well as an emaciated, wrinkled appearance. But those who have truly distorted views don't see themselves that way.

Exploding the myths about weight

Weight obsession is hardly a new thing in American culture. Since the early years of the 20th century, the public has been urged to "reduce." Some ads in lady's magazines of the time even promoted weight-reducing devices, but the ideal image of womanhood was still well-rounded. The Gibson girl of about 100 years ago was presented in the print media of the day as tall, gracefully vigorous, and solidly elegant, with softly rounded cheeks and chin. She was the last substantial-looking female Americans were encouraged to emulate. Very shortly afterward, the ideal image became that of the flapper, whose thin, hipless shape may have been the precursor to the "heroin chic" of the late 1990s.

During the 1940s, concern over obesity grew as a real public health problem, thanks to the nation's overabundance of food and the availability of labor-saving devices. At this time the pressure to slim down increased. Life insurance companies began publishing lists of ideal weights.

This is not to say that obesity is not a problem: It is one of the leading health risks for Americans and Westerners, in general. However, the hype about being "overweight" has led Americans to spend $33 billion on diet-related products—a threefold increase over two decades—while the average weight of the adult population is steadily rising. This should be a clue that common ideas about "ideal" weights are out of whack.

Unofficially... University of Toronto researchers weighed groups of dieters and nondieters. They then told the people within these groups that they weighed 5 pounds more or 5 pounds less than their actual weights. Dieters who believed that they had gained weight experienced a worsening of mood that led them to overeat.

Destroying distorted body images

Commercial artists and others in the magazine and catalog industries know that virtually every representation of the human body on the printed page is trimmed and retouched to "perfection." In the film and video industries, lighting and camera angles have always been the arts that make people look slimmer. These projections are not real, but it's almost impossible to separate idealized images from reality. It's especially hard for some young people.

A recent survey by the About-Face organization (a nonprofit group devoted to studying the impact of the meida on distorted body image and distorted eating), found that girls as young as age 8 consider themselves too fat compared to images of girls and women in style magazines—this is only the latest in a series of studies and observations that connect body image to marketing efforts. Researchers at About-Face have found that the media reflect images of thinness and link them to symbols of prestige, happiness, love, and success for women. Here are a few other findings from About-Face:

- Sixty-nine percent of female television characters are thin; only 5 percent are overweight.

- The average person sees between 400 and 600 advertisements per day; that is 40 million to 50 million by the time he is 60 years old.

- The incidence of anorexia nervosa among 10- to 19-year-old girls parallels the change in fashion from plumper to thinner models and points to a correlation between cultural acceptance of idealized, thin body images and high rates of anorexia nervosa.

- People who were exposed to slides of thin models consequently expressed lower self-evaluations than subjects who did not see the slides.

Harvard University mental health researchers have also found that eating disorders can be regarded as a cultural phenomenon and a social problem, noting that in this country women are becoming heavier with each generation, while the body presented as ideal for health or beauty becomes slimmer. As a possible result of this, the Harvard report finds the following:

- More than half of American women say they are on a diet.

- Of fifth- to eighth-grade girls, 31 percent said they were dieting, 9 percent said they some-times fasted, and 5 percent had deliberately induced vomiting.

- In 1950, 7 percent of men and 14 percent of women said they were trying to lose weight. In the early 1990s, 37 percent of men and 52 per-cent of women thought they were overweight; 24 percent of men and 40 percent of women said they were dieting.

And then there are the diet ads and infomer-cials—the constant barrage of "self-improvement" messages that remind the audience that they *could* be better. These ads even appear in banners on resource pages for eating-disorder information on the Internet! And fine print discourages the audi-ence from reading important information such as, "Not a typical result." No one is ever encouraged to think that if the advertised diets really worked, there would be no need for more ads or products.

Unofficially... The average weight of Miss America winners has been declin-ing steadily since the pageant was initiated.

Watch Out!
A survey of *Essence* magazine's African American readers found levels of abnormal eating attitudes and body dissatisfaction that were at least as high as a similar survey of Caucasian women.

Equal opportunity impact

About-Face has studied the impact of images on a diverse audience. Until recently, eating disorders were considered a white, middle- and upper-class disease. Increasingly, women of color are coming forward with eating disorders, a fact that parallels the appearance of more slender models in black media, the organization notes. The group is also tracking media images around the world and has found similar parallels in Asia and South America. Global media, it seems, is mainstreaming women around the world into the Western beauty myth, which has been so heavily influenced by American media standards of what is "attractive."

Not every victim of an eating disorder is female. At least 1 out of every 10 people who has an eating disorder is a man or a boy who may be just as susceptible to media ideals as his female counterpart. As with women, the ideal male body image has changed over time and has become slimmer and more muscular. Remember that at least half of those bodies on *Baywatch* are male.

Never too young to feel "too fat"

Social scientists are finding distorted eating patterns in increasingly younger children. They also link eating disorders to dieting, which is also occurring at younger ages. One study found that 5 percent of teenage girls reported binge eating and purging by age 16—most of them began dieting at a younger age. In other words, young people connect self-worth with shape and size—and their dissatisfaction with their shape and size has a negative effect on other important areas of their lives, beginning at an early age.

COMPARISONS AND CONTRASTS:
IDEAL VERSUS REAL PEOPLE

33–23–33 = Average measurements of a contemporary fashion model

as compared with:

36–18–33 = Projected measurements of a Barbie doll, in inches, if she was a full-size woman

---

5 feet, 4 inches / 142 = Average height and weight of an American woman

as compared with:

5 feet, 9 inches / 110 = Average height and weight of a model

---

33% of American women wear a size 16 or larger

80% of American women diet at some point

25% of American men diet at some point

50% of American women are on a diet at any one time

50% of 9-year-old girls have dieted at some point

10% of teenagers with eating disorders are boys

Body-image distortion affects young boys as well as girls. A mismatch of body image and reality begins at a surprisingly early age for both boys and girls. In a study of children aged 8–10, approximately half the girls and one third of the boys were dissatisfied with their size. However, most of the dissatisfied girls wanted to be thinner, while about an equal number of dissatisfied boys wanted to be heavier. No matter what the actual size of these children, approximately half of the girls and one third of the boys chose a slimmer body.

When the mirror lies: Negative body image

The dissonance between the reflection in the mirror and the glossy, airbrushed photos in major

Watch Out!
Obesity in children can be a danger sign. It may indicate diabetes or reflect other physical or emotional health problems. On the other hand, it may simply be a developmental phase that should be analyzed by a physician.

magazines is an indicator that people who have serious eating disorders—and many more whose thinking about weight is just somewhat disordered—internalize dissatisfactions with their actual appearance.

When asked to express what these people think of themselves, their thoughts sound like this:

> "I think I'm fat.... I'm a horrible person....
> I must deserve this.... It's my own fault....
> My problems don't matter.... Others don't
> deserve an eating disorder, but I'm
> different...."

Body-image disturbance is a problem both in how people see their bodies and in the way they think and feel about what their *perceptions* mean. For instance, a woman might think her hips are too large, but in the greater scheme of things, big hips might not mean that much to her. She might like other things about her body, so it isn't important to her that her hips are "too large." Another woman, on the other hand, also might think that her hips are too large, but unlike the first woman, she concludes that no one will ever be attracted to her, that she's a loser, that other people are superior, and so on. So, the problem is not just how people see themselves, but the feelings and meanings they attach to what they see.

It is all too common for people living with anorexia and bulimia to have mild to severely distorted perceptions of themselves. What they see in the mirror doesn't reflect reality, and when they compare their physical attributes or personalities to others, they are extremely critical of themselves. A person suffering from anorexia or bulimia may see another person and think, "I wish I could be as skinny as her," when in reality, she may be thinner. She may wish to be as smart, as funny, or as compassionate as another person, while having all those qualities herself. The bottom line is that she cannot see her own good traits because of low self-esteem.

Telltale signs

Because shape-consciousness pervades Western culture, people who are truly compulsive may be able to hide their obsessions. But experts can clearly see signs of overconcern with image. For example, it is a common practice for the overly body-conscious to wear baggy, layered clothing. This not only reflects dissatisfaction with one's appearance, but it also serves to hide any radical loss of weight. Over-exercising is another indicator that someone may be overly concerned with body image. People who exercise solely for good health work out every other day, while those who are obsessed with body image exercise for long periods every day. (See Chapter 7, "Exercise Disorders," for more details about compulsive exercising.)

It can be argued that overexercise is often stimulated by the media. The number of exercise programs on television and the sale of exercise videos has increased radically in the last decade. At the same time, the body shapes promoted by these shows and tapes are largely unattainable under normal life conditions.

Reality check

Eating disorder specialists believe a direct connection exists between a confused or distorted body image and eating disorders.

Although most American women have some body image distortion, it gets out of control for some women. Counselors point to telltale behaviors

Moneysaver
Charting your responses to images of yourself can help you decide if a diet is really necessary. For example, if one mirror-check gets an "I'm fat and ugly" response and the very next rates a "Not too bad," this may be a sign that the image you see is more a reflection of an inner feeling than an outward reality. Forget the diet.

such as repetitive body checking. Many of us might not be able to pass a mirror or window without checking our hair, teeth, or overall appearance, but a person with a body image disturbance may pay special attention to how fat or how flat his stomach appears over the course of the day. A woman with a distorted self-image might spend two angry and despairing hours every morning trying to find an outfit that doesn't make her "look fat," when she may look fine in all of them.

It also has been shown that how we feel affects how we see ourselves. People whose self-esteem is high tend to think they look better than perhaps they do. Body image is a good indicator of both physical and mental well-being. A severely distorted body image can be an indication of an eating disorder.

The image/reality conflict probably affects most people in our culture by instilling at least a small measure of dissatisfaction with the difference between the way we look and the beautiful-body images that surround us. However, discrepancies between these body images can be devastating to anyone who has the potential for an eating disorder and who feels driven to excessive efforts to match an unrealistic ideal.

Just the facts

- The influence of mass media on how we perceive images of the body has a demonstrable effect on how we feel about our own bodies.

- The ideal body types promoted by the media are far slimmer and leaner than normal and may not even be healthy for real people.

- In recent decades, the weight of people depicted as "ideal" in media images has actually declined steadily. As a result of this, more money has been lavished on diet and exercise, while the weight of the average person has actually increased.

- Distorted body images can start very early in life and affect children's feelings about themselves

- A direct connection exists between body image distortion and the severity of an eating disorder

Mixed messages about food, and where
they come from ▪ Unhealthy eating
patterns ▪ How dieting triggers food disorders
▪ Why eating disorders are not about food
▪ The "normalcy" dilemma

Our Relationship with Food

Chapter 3

O ur relationship with food should be as simple as taking in and expending the amount of fuel we need to thrive and enjoy life. But the fact is that relating to food is not that simple for anyone, least of all those who are predisposed to eating disorders.

This chapter and the previous one focus on two elements that characterize all disordered eating: troubled relationships with food and misperceptions of body image. The fact that these characteristics occur in the context of a more general state of food confusion only worsens their effect.

Mixed messages about food

Consider these apparently contradictory facts:

In the United States, retail food stores are a $450 billion industry. The diet and weight-loss industry generates some $33 billion. At the same time, approximately 25 percent of men and 45 percent of women are trying to lose weight, according to the American Dietetic Association.

Magazines that feature "super diets" and "thigh reduction" are supported by advertisements for chocolate cake. We find nothing odd about snacking in front of television advertisements that sell exercise machines and memberships to weight-loss organizations. And what about all those Sunday afternoons spent in sports bars, watching the game while drinking beer and eating chips and sandwiches? Even Americans who consider themselves "normal" eaters have something of a confused—if not disordered—relationship with food.

Market-driven eating

To say that those of us who live in a Western culture receive mixed messages about food is to dramatically understate the powerful contradictions between the informational and emotional messages we receive from sources all around us, whether it's the mass media or those nearest and dearest to us.

Food brings us comfort, but too much of this kind of comfort brings the social *discomfort* of being "too fat" by media-ruled standards. Fitness carries as high a value in our culture as leanness, but carry *it* too far and it's impossible to be truly "fit."

Food gives us fuel to energize the activities of life. In cultures that are closer to nature than ours, the only concern is to get enough food to carry on with life. In modern societies, on the other hand, the balance between food and energy would seem to be way out of sync.

As necessary as it is for *us* to eat, it's even more necessary to consume enough to keep the food industry humming. So advertisers and marketers urge us to buy and eat. The irony, of course, is that they use ads filled with skinny models to motivate us to do just that. No wonder we feel compelled to diet.

Watch Out!
"Examine closely your dreams and goals for your children," urges Dr. Michael Levine of the Eating Disorders Awareness Project. "Decide what you can do to reduce the vilification of overweight and the glorification of slenderness."

This is not to say that modern America invented eating disorders, but it would be hard to find anyone in any contemporary Western culture who hasn't been on some kind of diet or exercise program.

Parents absorb all the marketing hype and advertising messages along with everyone else, of course. Without being aware of it, they pass these messages along to their children, reinforcing what their children have already received. Even families that have no serious food-related neurosis may be awash in food-related misinformation and confusion: "A chubby baby is a happy baby," but "slender is good," "Kids *like* sweet foods." "Plates should be cleaned."

Parents encourage and sometimes even force kids to eat, and then they either recoil in horror when their children eat too much and get fat, or express bewilderment when kids use noneating as a way of rebelling.

Parents who have absorbed the mass-market message that slim is good will casually comment on their children's friends: "He's a nice-looking boy" (if he's slim). Or, "He's a real roly-poly!"(if he's not). When parents consider their children as extensions of themselves and their egos—as so often is the case—they naturally want Junior to "look good" (slim, in other words).

So maybe it's little wonder that children as young as 8 have started dieting, and that a majority of all children in the United States have been on some kind of reducing diet by the time they've reached fourth grade.

Disordered eating patterns

In sum, the culture gives everyone mixed messages about food, urging all of us to eat but chastising us

Bright Idea
Parents can be role models for their children by avoiding a focus on dieting and overexercising. By setting a good example, they may also do themselves a favor.

for not being lean. This may be one reason why there are so many people who do not have a clinical eating disorder but who struggle with disordered eating nonetheless. These "normal" eaters realize that they are *not* eating like a "normal person." Very often, they can be just as obsessed with thoughts of food as the person who has been clinically diagnosed with an eating disorder.

Using food as a crutch

Food is supposed to make people feel good, we're told. And it does: Experience shows that life looks and feels better on a full stomach. Brain function is better, too. The hypothalamus sends out "feel-good" hormones, so it's natural that people might use food to get them through stressful or unhappy times.

All it takes is a quick look at our sped-up society to get an idea of the negative impact our eating habits can have—even on "normal" people. Too little time to eat and too much junk food eaten on the run—combined with over-nervous activity and lack of nutrition—produces fatigue, which in turn causes more disordered eating.

People who have anorectic tendencies feel that the world is spinning out of control and have learned that one thing they *can* control in life is their food intake. Restricting food puts them back in control; if the pace of life is overwhelming, not eating ultimately numbs their feelings of inadequacy and their inability to "keep up." Thus not eating becomes a crutch and, as we'll see later, a coping mechanism.

Using food as a defense

Eating is a way to take care of ourselves and to feel good. That's true—and it's a truth that is confirmed repeatedly by certain media messages. But, again,

Unofficially...
Some people who have food obsessions think of food nearly 75 percent of the day.

going too far in the feel-good department makes us fat, and in our culture being fat is a sign of *not* being good.

Food very often becomes a weapon when it's aimed at someone nearby who is getting in the way of a person's goals: "I would have been promoted if I didn't have this extra weight," the anger-filled husband tells his wife. "And if you didn't keep cooking those high-calorie meals, I wouldn't weigh so much!"

A child may spit out spinach at a well-meaning parent, or an older child may stop eating as a way to get back at a parent who may or may *not* mean well. A 12-year-old girl whose mother has always called her "chubby" may eat only grapefruit—until the divorced Dad steps in to rescue the situation (giving the daughter the extra bonus of Dad's attention).

As they head toward adulthood and begin to feel that they are failing various reality checks, many children use food as a weapon against themselves. Whether they take an eating disorder to the extreme that it threatens their health, this problem restricts their lives radically. Eating disorders limit social life when children no longer go out to eat or skip outings because they feel fat. The amount of mental energy and time spent thinking about food and body issues detracts from other areas of their lives as well.

How dieting triggers food disorders

The more Americans diet, the less effect it seems to have. Despite all the dieting and money spent on weight-loss products, programs, and equipment, the average weight is rising. In fact our collective obsession with getting thinner may be contributing to our increasing obesity, especially now that it has been demonstrated that constant dieting leads to

Moneysaver
Experts say that dieting causes overeating by setting up the body to increase food intake sooner or later. So why not save the money spent on diet foods and books, and avoid diets? There *are* other ways to maintain a healthy balance.

"

I hadn't really meant to lose 15 pounds in three weeks, but once they were off, I was determined above all else not to put them back on.
—A high school student who found herslef caught in an eating disorder spiral

"

increases in weight. According to the American Dietetics Association, weight cycling—or "yo-yo-ing"—may be more harmful than carrying a few extra pounds of body weight. The cycle of repeatedly losing and regaining weight makes weight management more difficult over the long run and may even increase the risk for some health problems. Yet people keep dieting.

Counselors at New York University's Counseling Center explain to their clients who have eating disorders that an adverse effect of dieting can be bingeing, which is dangerous in itself and which counteracts any "success" one may have achieved with a diet. This is how they explain the process, using Dr. Christopher Fairburn's model:

- There are three forms of dieting:

    1. Avoiding eating for long periods of time (in other words, starving, which may lead to bingeing)

    2. Avoiding eating certain types of food (cravings for these foods may lead to bingeing)

    3. Restricting the total amount of food eaten (starving, which, again, may lead to bingeing)

- People develop dietary rules about what they should and should not eat that become increasingly rigid and extreme, as well as impossible to obey, particularly in times of stress. Deviations from these rules are viewed as evidence of poor self-control rather than proof that the rules themselves are faulty. This can lead to abandoning all control: "I broke my diet, so I might as well binge. I'll start again tomorrow."

- Once control is abandoned, other factors contribute to overeating: pleasure in eating forbidden foods, distraction from current problems, and temporary relief from depression and anxiety.

How the obsession spreads

People who are susceptible to eating disorders take cultural messages that "slim is good" and that "successful people are thin" to the extreme.

They might spend most of their waking hours thinking about food or in a quest for food. Their pursuit of thinness or their obsession with food drives them to punish their bodies through binge eating, bingeing and purging, or starvation.

This confusion between worth and body shape is triggered by the culture that surrounds us, and it appears that the American preoccupation with weight may be spreading.

As the world becomes a global village connected by CNN and the Internet, our values are having an impact on previously isolated communities. The marketing that previously had affected only affluent, technologically sophisticated societies is sneaking into older, once tradition-bound societies. For example, eating disorders were very rare in Asia until recently, when Western influence began portraying images of slender young immigrant women who had adopted the "American way of dieting."

Researchers studying women who have immigrated to the United States from other cultures find that they adapt fairly quickly to the weight-management attitudes of our culture and decide that they must diet because they are "too fat."

Four degrees of separation

What makes disordered eating all the more complicated is that we *do* have to eat. People whose

Timesaver
Women's weight normally goes up or down by about 6 pounds, regardless of food intake. Water retention, bowel movements, menstrual cycle—all have an effect on weight and have nothing to do with food intake. Don't conclude that a two pound weight gain indicates a need to diet. Wait two weeks to see if the gain is consistent before changing food habits.

compulsions involve alcohol, gambling, or addictive drugs may have a tough time breaking free of them; but when they do, they stop completely. People who act compulsively with food have a trickier time: They have to eat *something*. They can't stay away from food altogether. If they don't eat, they'll eventually die.

Disordered eating is one span in the same continuum that *begins* with "normal" behavior. For example:

- The "normal" or typical individual who has a healthy approach to food eats at appropriate times (that is, when he is hungry) and stops when he is full. He gets enough exercise during the day to keep his system in order, and he may not weigh himself except when having physical checkups.

- The "health-conscious" individual in today's society is careful to concentrate on foods that are known to be healthy. She makes selections from the food guide pyramid and avoids foods that might endanger her health. She makes a special effort to get exercise at least three times a week and may weigh herself once every week or two.

- The "chronic dieter" keeps careful track of foods, which he selects from a limited list. He focuses on those that will help him lose weight and avoids those that might cause weight gain. Chronic dieters conscientiously exercise at least once or twice a day and weigh themselves daily.

- The person who has a food disorder, such as anorexia nervosa, eats only a few low-calorie foods and considers all others "dangerous." She exercises many hours every day and weighs herself frequently.

Watch Out!
Chronic dieting can stop the sensation of hunger, so people who need to get their eating back on track should use a clock as a cue to eat. The sensation of hunger will return after a more regular pattern of eating has been established.

The hidden game plan:
It's not about food

Given the fact that disordered thinking about food and body image can be so gradual, pervasive, and self-destructive, it is not surprising to learn from psychologists that eating disorders are *not* about food. They are about emotions—especially anger—turned inward.

Anger that fuels serious and potentially deadly eating disorders is often turned against the world or a family that has spun out of control. It might begin as an effort to bring some order to the maddening confusion: "I have the power to fix this." It might begin as anger turned against parents whose demands can never be met and which fosters an "I'll show you how good I can be" effort that results in slow suicide.

Inward-turned anger can follow a progression that seems to make a certain kind of sense—at least at first. The (unconscious) mental monologue might sound like this, over a period of time:

- "I'm not good enough—in fact, I am *so* not good that I hate myself."

- "I can make myself better by shaping up with 'good' food and exercise."

- "Exercise and eating right is working—but not enough. I *really* must be a loser.... If I could just get control!"

- "Now I'm eating *only* good foods and exercising for hours every day, but it feels good to deprive myself, so I'll do it even more."

- "I am *really* worthless! I hate myself so much that I'm going to punish myself. Here are the rules, you undisciplined loser: No food until you shape up!"

Unofficially...
If a person who
has anorexia or
bulimia treated a
child the same
way she treats
herself, she
could be arrested
for abuse or
neglect.

Of course, the "shape up" never comes because the person's distorted thinking inevitably leads to starvation, binge eating, and more self-hate. The starving individual feels worse emotionally as his body's chemical balance shifts into "depression" mode. Thus the cycle reinforces itself. The ultimate result of inward-directed anger is self-destruction.

The psychological aspect of disordered eating is intense. Indeed, it is not unlike those that underlie other self-destructive behaviors such as alcoholism, drug addiction, or suicidal syndromes. In this case, food is the chosen tool.

Why food?

Why one person chooses food as a weapon rather than alcohol, pills, a needle, or a gun is not known precisely, except that food is legal, available, and socially acceptable.

It is the very innocuous nature of the substance—compared to alcohol or drugs, for instance—that makes eating disorders so insidious. Given the fact that everyone has to eat and that most people today want to "eat healthy" and "lose weight," a destructive eating pattern may be well underway before anyone (including the sufferer) realizes what's going on.

Drawing the line

A turn of the millennium American may easily develop eating patterns that include chronic dieting, overexercise, and unbalanced nutrition largely because of mistaken beliefs about what is "healthy" and what a "normal" weight should be.

"Drawing a line between eating disorders and the consequences of 'normal,' socially approved dieting is not easy," a Harvard University report notes. If food brings so much confusion to the mainstream of modern culture, it's hardly any wonder that it can create such havoc in the lives and bodies of people whose emotional state is already disordered. People who are susceptible to eating disorders carry "normal" patterns to extremes in anorexia and bulimia.

What's surprising is how widely accepted some disordered eating habits are by people who would not consider themselves anything other than normal.

While we might generally agree that a skeletal young woman who forces herself to vomit after every meal has a serious problem, it may be harder to see an eating disorder at work in a normal everyday scenario, such as any one of these:

- A woman who once had bulimia and whose set point (that is, her natural weight) is higher than the height-weight charts, diets constantly to keep her weight below her natural level:

  Unless she can maintain an appropriate weight without dieting, her eating disorder will persist.

- A teenage girl starts to smoke cigarettes:

  Surveys indicate that the main motive for smoking in adolescent girls is weight control.

- A 65-year-old man dies from what appears to be malnutrition, despite the fact that he lives in comfortable surroundings:

  Older adults show a surprisingly high rate of eating disorders, which are much more likely to cause death, particularly in men.

- A well-muscled male college athlete collapses on the playing field:

  A particularly dangerous pattern occurs in young men who want to look both lean and muscular: They combine radical dieting with steroids.

Bright Idea
To zero in on Americans' conflicting relationship with food, take a close look at the magazines that are most often found on racks by the checkout counters in supermarkets (where else?). Study the ads for food, and study the articles—the majority of which are about food, dieting, and exercise—for photos of attractive, slim women. Is there anything confusing about these juxtapositions?

Unofficially...
When passing a mirror or a shop window, people with body-image distortions tend to look at the reflection of their bellies first. In private, they focus on the mirror's reflection of the parts of their bodies they consider fattest.

Timesaver
Walk down the aisles of the grocery store you shop in most often. Make a list of foods you don't eat—and why. Which of the foods are most "safe" for you? Which are "unsafe"? You may be surprised by what is brought into focus by this exercise. The length of your list and the items on it may point to an incipient eating disorder.

Certainly, a major difference exists between people who truly have life- or health-threatening eating disorders and people in the mainstream whose patterns of eating are disordered to one degree or another. But the very fact that so many people in our society have even a somewhat distorted relationship with food is an indication of how serious and widespread the situation is.

Just the facts

- People in modern Western cultures automatically face confusion about food and eating habits because of the proliferation of commercial messages about diet.

- Parents who may have sound motives can nevertheless instill harmful attitudes about food in their children.

- Eating disorders are more about anger turned inward than they are about food.

- The most common trigger for an eating disorder is a weight-loss diet.

- In the context of "normal" cultural confusions about food, a serious eating disorder may be difficult to spot.

Eating Disorders

GET THE SCOOP ON...
Defining anorexia nervosa? ▪ What anorexia
looks and feels like ▪ Warning signs ▪ Targets of
anorexia ▪ Personal profiles

PART II

Chapter 4

Anorexia Nervosa

The term *anorexia* means an absence of eating. *Nervosa* refers to the psychological source of the condition, from the Latin word meaning "nervous." Put the words together, and they describe a psychologically irrational, self-destructive pattern of starvation. The term is so prevalent today that it is often loosely applied to any kind of underweight condition, but anorexia has very specific symptoms.

The doctors' definition
As explained by the National Institutes of Mental Health, anorexia nervosa is an emotional weight-loss disorder characterized by physical, social, and psychological symptoms. Loss of weight to unhealthy levels is achieved by a variety of compulsive behaviors.

According to the American Psychiatric Association, clinical anorexia is diagnosed when weight has fallen to 15 percent below the normal range and, in the case of a woman, lack of menstruation for at least three months.

More detailed professional descriptions include the refusal to maintain body weight at or above a minimally normal weight for age and height, an intense fear of gaining weight, and a firm sense of "being fat" no matter what the actual weight.

It is critically important to understand that anorexia nervosa is a progressive disorder. In other words, without treatment, it will only get worse and may even lead to death. Consequently, professionals err on the side of caution when they suspect anorexia.

Most people who have eating problems don't meet the full criteria of anorexia. Nevertheless, they have an eating disorder that has *anorectic characteristics*. The official diagnosis for this is: "Eating Disorder, Not Otherwise Specified with Anorectic Features." Therefore, these people have many of the same physical, emotional, and social concerns as someone who has anorexia and need treatment.

Two kinds of anorexia exist now. One form involves people who restrict their food; the other includes those who binge-eat and purge. In other words, a person can meet all four of the diagnostic criteria but also binge and purge and still have anorexia (see the box, "Diagnostic Criteria for Anorexia," on the next page). Some specialists refer to purging as a progression of anorexia into bulimia. People who have anorexia report discovering purging as an additional way to control their weight. In other words, anorexia is not just for people who restrict their food anymore.

What anorexia looks like

In the extreme phase of the disorder, people who have anorexia look emaciated, with dry, sallow skin, brittle nails and thin hair. Their limbs are often covered with a fine downy hair called lanugo. But this is

Watch Out!
Doctors stress that most people who have eating disorders do not display all symptoms of anorexia. So, someone with a partial set of symptoms—or only a hint of them—would be wise to investigate further because early treatment is key to success.

Diagnostic criteria for anorexia

1. Refusal to maintain normal body weight (85 percent of expected weight or less)

2. Intense fear of gaining weight

3. Body image distortion

4. Amenorrhea (absence of menstrual period) for three months (unless they are on birth control pills, in which case menstruation may continue)

---

the extreme: Doctors note that many people who have anorexia can't be identified by their appearance.

Many people who have anorexia or anorectic features appear to be as "normal" as the next person. Therefore, it's important to stress that you can't necessarily identify someone who has anorexia simply by looking at her.

Even before the disorder has progressed to the extremes of starvation, people who have anorexia display some common characteristics. For example, they tend to be perfectionists who set unrealistically high expectations for themselves in many areas of their lives. These expectations often lead to stress, low self-esteem, and loss of control. For people who have anorexia, restricting what they eat is a way to feel in control.

What anorexia often looks like to an observer is perhaps little more than a set of eccentric food rituals such as cutting and dicing food into small pieces, arranging food in a particular way on the plate, and chewing a certain number of times before swallowing. Other habits might include collecting recipes and food coupons; obsessively counting calories;

cooking and baking for others; hoarding and eating food secretly; and being preoccupied constantly with food, weight, and body size and shape. People who have eating disorders tend to wear layered, loose-fitting clothes to conceal the changing shape of their bodies, and they demonstrate excessive activity, restlessness, and insomnia.

Many women whose weights are normal severely restrict their intake of food. These women have amenorrhea, suffer from body image distortion, and are fearful of weight gain. Their metabolism has slowed down so much that they're able to maintain their weight on very few calories. This occurrence of anorectic features along with normal body weight is becoming more common. It can be dangerously deceptive because many doctors who have not been educated in eating disorders assume that there is no problem if a woman's weight is normal. However, there may be a very serious problem, despite what the scale says.

What anorexia feels like

Most people who have anorexia initially deny it, despite medical tests that reveal telltale symptoms. Many continue to deny it even when they must be hospitalized to prevent possible permanent damage or even death from starvation. Dehydration causes excessive thirst and constipation, and reduced body fat leads to lowered body temperature and the inability to withstand cold. People who have anorexia also experience reduced muscle mass and light-headedness. While growing increasingly weak, they may refuse to admit that anything is wrong. Starvation can lead to poor brain function, which muddles thinking and makes dealing with reality that much more of a challenge. Starvation, especially when done by purging, can also deplete the body of

---

Physical Effects of Severe Dieting

Some of the effects of severe dieting are listed here. However, not all of them need to be apparent for dieting to have a destructive effect on the body.

1. Slowed metabolism

2. Emaciated appearance

3. Dry, sometimes yellowish skin

4. Blood pressure changes

5. Decreased heart rate and body temperature

6. Decrease in bone density

7. Shrinkage of brain tissue

8. Fluid and electrolyte problems; gastrointestinal, cardiac, and menstrual complications

9. Drowsiness and lethargy

10. Swelling in lower extremities

---

potassium and other electrolytes, the substances that transmit nerve impulses within the body. Without these signals, organs—including the heart—function poorly and may come to a complete halt.

A person who has anorexia may become hyperactive and dizzy, and may feel a "buzz" at all times. He may feel depressed, irritable, and withdrawn and may be prone to compulsive rituals, such as dividing food into tiny portions or placing food in small jars and lining them up.

Physical realities

The physical consequences of anorexia are not just feeling sick, however: Internal deterioration is

Unofficially...
People who have anorexia usually deny having a problem, saying that everything is under control. They claim that the people who are trying to help them only want to make them fat.

pervasive. For example, the level of female hormones in the blood falls drastically, resulting in delayed sexual development. Heart rate and blood pressure drop dangerously low, and loss of potassium in the blood may cause irregular heart rhythms. Muscles atrophy or waste away, resulting in weakness and loss of muscle function. Loss of bone calcium leads to osteoporosis and brittle bones that are prone to breakage. Over a 10-year period, about 5 percent of women who suffer from anorexia will die, mainly from infections or cardiac failure.

Despite the fact that anorexia poses serious health risks, people who have anorexia use starvation as an attempt to gain control and cope with life's stresses even as starvation causes the gradual deterioration and eventual systemwide failure of the body.

Personal effects

The only people who truly know how it feels to have anorexia are those who have lived through it:

> "This is what it's like to live an anorexic life," says Judy. "Cold all the time, people watching you strangely, feeling like nothing matters but your weight, hating the thought of eating 'unsafe foods.'"

> Colleen recounts the voices of an eating disorder that say: "You're fat," "You're disgusting," "You don't deserve to eat," "You're worthless," and "You deserve to die."

Anorexia is a never-ending monologue that plays inside the mind from the minute the person who has it wakes up until the minute she falls asleep. The voices encourage their victims to continue to abuse their bodies through starvation, bingeing, purging, and other dangerous methods of weight control that can bring them to the brink of death. As one young woman put it:

> "They convince us that we are worthless, unlovable, fat, ugly, disgusting, hopeless, and worse. They convince us that the world would be better off without us and that we deserve to die. They will tell you that no one will love you if you gain weight. These voices are very powerful, and their ultimate goal is to destroy you."

But anorexia need not be so dramatic to still be painfully real and potentially dangerous. For example, a young 5-foot-5-inch woman who eats mostly salads, some tuna fish, and bananas may have managed to keep her weight at 122 pounds. That's "normal" by the charts, but she may struggle constantly to lose more weight and severely restrict her diet.

When it isn't anorexia

From the previous descriptions, it should be clear that worrying about weight gain or overspending on exercise equipment is not a sign of a serious eating disorder. When researchers study disordered eating, they eliminate subjects who are temporarily dieting or fasting. While it might be healthier to be more accepting of one's body, this kind of behavior usually doesn't qualify as "disordered."

Sometimes it is hard to tell when an eating problem has crossed the line and become a serious problem. The solution is to check any suspicions with a professional because even mild symptoms can lead to bigger ones. Some specialists in eating disorders label any kind of diet as "abnormal eating," but in today's culture, dieting is so widespread that it is simply impractical to call any sort of focus on eating "disordered." Indeed, it can be very hard to tell

Moneysaver
Seek early treatment of anorexia, even if you only suspect that you have it. Treatment of full-blown anorexia can be lengthy and extremely costly. Many HMOs also resist paying for it.

when weight loss is normal and when it signals a disorder. For example, a young woman, who had just started a very stressful job straight out of college began to run 5 miles every night at the gym and ate only "healthy" food "to combat stress." Her weight dropped from 111 pounds to 93 pounds. After a routine checkup, her gynecologist sounded the alarm. The young woman insists that she eats, and her mother confirms that she eats pasta and bagels. The young woman denies that she has anorexia or any other concerns about eating. How do you tell? Who's right?

A couple of indicators can help clarify whether a person has an eating disorder or whether she has simply lost weight due to stress or some other temporary condition.

1. Is the person eating food from all food groups without anxiety? The young woman in the previous example has been told by her doctor that she needs to regain some weight for her health. How easy will it be for her to choose higher-fat, higher-calorie foods? Will she feel comfortable adding a slice of cheese or putting mayonnaise on a sandwich? Is she able to eat dessert on occasion? If she can eat a wide variety of foods from all food groups without anxiety, she probably doesn't have an eating disorder.

2. How rigid or flexible is the person about changing her behavior? The woman in this example was running 5 miles a day. Can she stop or reduce the number of miles she runs now that she knows that her health is at risk and that she needs to gain weight? Can she develop other methods of handling stress that don't result in weight loss?

If a person is eating a full range of foods without anxiety and is flexible about managing stress and other everyday challenges, she probably doesn't have an eating disorder.

Warning signs of anorexia

The line between healthy and disordered behavior is hazy, at best, but there are some red flags. Please note that *some* of the behaviors listed here may *not* be related to eating disorders at all. For example, we don't mean to suggest that if someone is a vegetarian, he has an eating disorder, but the elimination of one or more food groups from one's diet usually merits further inquiry.

1. Total elimination of a food group (or groups). Anyone can cut down on fats or red meat, but if a person eliminates all fat, meat, and dairy from her diet, it could be a warning sign of an eating disorder. When a doctor hears from a patient that she is a vegetarian, a vegan, or lactose-intolerant, or if she has food allergies, that doctor's antennae go up. When did the patient become one? Was it before or after eating became an issue?

2. Constant consumption of appetite suppressants. This includes hard candies, chewing gum, coffee, diet sodas, or cigarettes—all of which can suppress the appetite.

3. Fears or beliefs about food. For example, a cookie could be perceived as a "dangerous" substance; the very thought of eating pasta with cream sauce could be "nightmarish."

4. Preoccupation with the appearance of the body. This also includes overconcern about a particular part of the body.

5. Hours of searching for outfits that don't "make" one look "fat."

6. Compulsive exercising, even during sickness, in all kinds of weather, or at any time of the day or night.

7. Avoidance of plans involving meals or last-minute cancellations of lunch or dinner dates.

8. Sudden cessation of alcohol consumption because of the empty calories.

Again, these signs don't necessarily mean that someone has an eating disorder, but they might suggest there's a problem. It is very important to pay attention to even a few symptoms because (1) they *can* mark the beginning of an eating disorder, and (2) getting treatment early improves a prognosis.

Who has anorexia?

The stereotype of the person who has anorexia is young, white, female, and upper-middle-class. But demographics don't tell the whole story, even if most of the approximately 7 million cases of anorexia in the United States occur in women under the age of 35. Ten percent are men, however, and researchers are finding increasing numbers of older and even elderly sufferers.

Psychological profile

The classic psychological profile of a person who has anorexia is of a young woman who is "too good to be true"—someone who seems to have her life successfully in order. Professionals at the Harvard University Eating Disorders Center who study the structure behind this facade see starvation as a form of self-punishment. Unconsciously, people who have anorexia may be trying to please their parents, who, they feel, *should* make the rules and *should* set guidelines for their behavior.

Sometimes they create parents in their minds whose rules they can obey and whom they can please by meeting all of their expectations. The bright, apparently well-adjusted 12-year-old daughter of a divorced working mother who lies awake fretting about homework and who eats only grapefruit and spinach may be taking her life into her own hands. She could be trying to make rules for herself when there's no one else to make them for her, while at the same time trying to get "perfect" enough to gain the positive attention of her distracted parent. This creates an almost unbearable tension.

Although some psychological theories hold that food control is a way for young girls to deal with the challenges and threats of sexuality and adult responsibilities, there are probably other psychological payoffs as well because so many people who have anorexia don't fit the young-girl model.

Self-starvation goes against our most basic instincts for self-preservation, so it must be driven by an extremely powerful dynamic. A pre-pubescent girl may be frightened by sex or by the idea of growing up at all. Therefore, she may severely restrict the amount of food she eats as an unconscious way of avoiding maturation. An older man might be faced with life challenges that seem overwhelming, such as the need to succeed as a professional or to cope with family crises that are out of his control. The restriction of food can be a way to insert control of some kind into an apparently uncontrollable life, while at the same time offering a potential escape from the demands that person finds impossible to meet.

I was unhappy in my new school in grade 9, and at about the same time my mother started reading up on low-fat cooking and healthy eating. Being something of a perfectionist, I read them all and decided that if low-fat is good, then no-fat is even better. I honestly did eat plenty—just nothing that contained more than a gram or two of fat. Anything fat-free was totally allowed. I was never happy with my body entirely.... I always thought my stomach needed to lose a little layer from it, and I always felt horrible about my gut after I overate. But besides the fact that I obsessed constantly about what I was allowed to eat, when I could eat, what I was going to eat, and what I was *not* allowed to eat, I was pretty normal. I just wouldn't touch fat. I was judging my self-worth based on what I ate and what I looked like.

—A college student describing the onset of anorexia

Watch Out!
Anna was a college student when her weight dropped so low that her mother could feel her bones when she hugged her. After Anna's friends came to visit her, they were so shocked by her appearance that they didn't say anything about it. Anna's reaction was, "See, Mom, I'm okay. They didn't notice a thing!"

There are more immediate payoffs as well: Not eating can be a way to express anger, get people to pay attention, or numb painful feelings.

It is even possible to experience pleasure by depriving oneself of the payoff of feeling good: The self becomes a hated object, so venting one's rage against it could be satisfying and gratifying. Expressing anger in this way is similar to the release of taking out frustration on a pillow, as if the pillow were the source of one's frustration. The mechanism is the same, but the hated object is the self. One young woman in her early 20s not only deprives herself of food, but she won't allow herself to wear her favorite sweater or earrings, or even to sit in a comfortable chair. For this young woman, self-deprivation is an emotional kick that feels too good to resist.

The family connection

Researchers have observed that anorexia seems to run in families: The mothers of women who have anorexia often have (or have had) the disorder themselves. But until recently, there has been doubt about whether the disorder itself is inherited or whether it simply comes from a specific kind of family environment. The National Eating Disorders Organization, for example, notes that "persons with a family history of mood disorders, chemical dependency, and/or eating disorders appear to be at higher risk for the development of eating disorders." But it is not clear which comes first, the eating disorder or the family dysfunction. Some surveys have found that people who have anorexia come from families whose lives are in turmoil. But anorexia itself can create turmoil.

Emotional components

Emotionally, anorexia seems to be driven by fear that the world is spinning out of control and requires restrictions to bring it under control again. Guilt, shame, and anger also appear to play a part. In addition, there is the overwhelming concern that if the "right" thing isn't done, disaster will strike. This response to imaginary fear accounts for the emotional rigidity that is so common in people who have anorexia.

As mentioned before, a person who has anorexia feels guilty and ashamed that she is simply not good enough; she thinks she doesn't meet her parents' expectations and can't succeed in life. Consequently,

Bright Idea
Praise for children's efforts, regardless of outcome, gives them the message that perfectionism isn't a requirement and that it's okay to make mistakes.

she chooses one area of her life she can manage and controls it to an extreme. However, her own standards of success are even higher than her parents'. Consequently, she can never be successful "enough" at controlling her life.

Anger comes into the mix from a variety of sources, even from the victim herself—for not being "perfect," for example—and it is directed at her family and society for not being "fair" in apparently demanding that she be "perfect." Because it may be too frightening to direct her anger at its source— her parents, for example—she turns the anger inward and uses food deprivation as a means to express it.

An emotionally distorted view of the world and a mistaken sense of a person's place in it may cause someone who has an eating disorder to withdraw from close interactions with others. His efforts to "protect" his own disordered food habits isolates him even further from open relationships with other people. Another sad irony—that anorexia is "designed" to make one perfect in society's eyes—is that it pulls its victims away from the very people they so desperately want to approach.

Two personal views

At 16, Sylvia, a young woman now in treatment for her disorder, says that her anorexia really kicked in either as a way to attract dates or to hide from them—or maybe both. Soon after the pounds started dropping off, her menstrual periods stopped. As anorexia tightened its grip, Sylvia became obsessed with dieting and food and developed strange eating rituals. Every day she weighed all the food she would eat on a kitchen scale, cutting solids into minuscule pieces and precisely measuring liquids. She would

---

Emotional Characteristics of Anorexia Nervosa

Distorted body image (feeling fat when one is actually thin)

Perfectionism

Low self-esteem

Difficulties with intimacy

Difficulty identifying and expressing feelings

Difficulty asking for help

Irritability

Difficulty concentrating

Anxiety—difficulty handling stress

Easily frustrated

"All or nothing" thinking

---

then put her daily ration into small containers and line them up in neat rows. She also exercised compulsively, even after she weakened and became faint. No one was able to convince Sylvia that she was in danger.

Finally, her doctor insisted that she be hospitalized and carefully monitored for treatment of her illness. Even there, she says, she secretly continued her exercise regimen in the bathroom.

John, another victim of an eating disorder, consistently responded, "Everything's under control" to a simple "How are you?"

As an overweight child, John had been alternately overfed and chastised for his weight by his mother; he had been put on high doses of "diet pills" in adolescence. As a young adult, he lost a dramatic amount of weight and struggled through most of his adulthood to maintain it. He measured and controlled every calorie he consumed—even to the point of using a computer program for the task.

Over the years his relationships crumbled, and he was irritable and unhappy most of the time. Still, he stayed skinny to the point of gauntness. Although John was never diagnosed with an eating disorder, his food restrictions and other symptoms qualified him as having one. A therapist once labeled him "depressive"—and he denied that, too. John has never sought (or felt the need for) treatment for his eating disorder, and throughout his life he has continued to pour emotional energy into controlling his weight rather than dealing with the external challenges that have proven so defeating.

Neither Sylvia nor John exemplifies the stereotypical version of "The Anorexia Story." Yet both illustrate how physical, emotional, and environmental factors contribute to the development of anorexia. And, of course, their stories illustrate all too clearly the devastating effects of this disorder on their lives.

Just the facts

- Anorexia can cause serious health problems—even death.

- People who have anorexia display certain common patterns of behavior.

- People who have anorexia rarely admit that they have a problem.

- The voices of anorexia say, "You're fat" and "You'll never be good enough."

- Anorexia nervosa must be treated and can be cured in most cases, but it is essential to intervene at the earliest possible time.

GET THE SCOOP ON...
Defining bulimia nervosa ▪ What bulimia
looks and feels like ▪ Telltale symptoms ▪ The
connection with anorexia ▪ Targets of bulimia
▪ Personal profiles

Bulimia Nervosa

Chapter 5

Bulimia, which means "oxlike hunger" in Greek, gets its name from the gorging phase of the disorder. People who have bulimia rigidly restrict or control their intake of food until they are no longer able to—then they gobble food in great volume. In an attempt to counteract the often huge intake of food and calories, they purge themselves.

This binge-purge pattern sets bulimia apart from anorexia. However, the purpose of bulimia, like anorexia, is to control weight within irrational limits—and like anorexia, the full name includes *nervosa*, which refers to the psychological aspect of the disease.

The doctors' definition

Bulimia was just recently identified and labeled as a specific disorder, in 1979. To diagnose bulimia, doctors look for a pattern of bingeing. This pattern involves eating a huge quantity of food and then purging, which involves getting rid of the consumed food in some fashion. These activities occur within

---

Criteria Used to Diagnose Bulimia

1. Recurrent episodes of binge eating ("binge" meaning eating an unusually large amount of food in less time than one might normally and having a sense of no control over eating during the episode)

2. Recurrent inappropriate compensatory behavior to prevent weight gain, such as self-induced vomiting; misuse of laxatives, diuretics, enemas or other medications; fasting; or excessive exercising

3. Binge and compensatory behaviors that occur at least twice a week for three months in a row

4. Self-evaluation that is unduly influenced by body shape and weight

---

the context of a fear of fatness, which motivates the restriction of food and nutritional intake. To fit the bulimia diagnosis, the person must have episodes that occur at least twice a week for three months. Common techniques for purging include self-induced vomiting; abuse of emetics, laxatives, and diuretics; fasting; and excessive exercise.

Although bulimia has been considered distinct from anorexia, it has recently become clear that many people who have anorexia progress to bulimia by adding purging to their weight-control behaviors when other techniques don't prove effective enough.

What bulimia looks like

Compared to people who have anorexia, people who have bulimia tend to be normal or slightly above normal weight. Because bulimia does involve some eating, weight loss is not so dramatic. As a result, people who might become concerned over the appearance of someone who has anorexia might not even be aware that someone else has bulimia. Bulimia often creates a chubby-cheeked (or "chipmunk") look, but only because vomiting enlarges salivary glands in the neck. People who have bulimia but who don't purge don't even show those small clues, and they tend to be closer to normal weight or slightly overweight. In sum, a person who has bulimia doesn't look much different from anyone else.

People who have bulimia and who purge tend to have lower body weights, more depression, and greater body distortion than people who do not purge. Also, they're more likely to have medical problems resulting from the purging itself.

The warning signs of bulimia

Although bulimia stems from circumstances similar to those of anorexia, it is associated with some particularly telltale signs. Bulimia also may be present if there are other characteristics, such as a preoccupation with body shape (especially in adolescent girls or young women).

- Lengthy visits to the bathroom after meals
- Mood swings
- Purchases of large amounts of food, which suddenly disappears
- Sudden, rapid consumption of large quantities of food
- Unusual swelling around the jaw

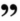

People might have guessed that I was unhappy, but they weren't likely to guess that I had bulimia. I was never especially thin or fat, my teeth never showed any scars, and I used eye drops and decongestants to hide the other signs.
—A young woman recovering from bulimia

Watch Out!
There are now two types of bulimia: purging, which involves vomiting or the use of laxatives, diuretics, and enemas to rid the body of food; and nonpurging, in which other compensatory behaviors, such as fasting or excessive exercising, are used without actual purging.

Watch Out!
Finding laxative
or diuretic wrap-
pers in the trash
while noting an
unexplained dis-
appearance of
food at home or
in a dormitory
should create a
suspicion of
bulimia.

These clues are particularly significant because weight loss is not always obvious in people who have bulimia.

The purging pattern

Purging can accomplish the weight loss sought by people who have bulimia, yet the motivation to purge must be very strong because it is a dangerous activity, no matter how it is done:

1. **Self-induced vomiting**—People sometimes use an emetic to induce vomiting or use their fingers to make themselves gag. After a while, some people who have bulimia are able to vomit by simply bending over the toilet. It is difficult to purge everything that has been ingested, however, because digestion has begun and some calories are absorbed before vomiting is initiated.

   Emetics such as ipecac are very dangerous and can cause nerve and muscle damage with frequent use. All vomiting can damage the esophagus, throat, and teeth.

   Vomiting generally produces a further breakdown in control over one's food intake, for it leads to more bingeing.

2. **Stimulant laxatives**—Stimulant laxatives flush out the large colon. However, all calories are absorbed in the *small* colon, making the use of stimulant laxatives an ineffective way to purge. Frequent use of laxatives may decrease bowel effectiveness, but some prefer it to vomiting.

3. **Diuretics**—Water pills reduce water weight but have no effect on calories or body fat. Ironically, the habitual use of diuretics produces *more* fluids in the body, which can result in water retention and possibly swelling of extremities, such as hands and feet.

Strategies to Reduce Bingeing

The key to getting free of "the bulimia cycle" is to eliminate dieting and to not let yourself get too hungry:

1. Eat every three hours to prevent hunger.

2. Eat from individual serving cartons—that is, do not buy a half gallon of ice cream; rather, eat individual serving portions.

3. After preparing a meal and filling your plate, put away the leftovers, in the freezer if necessary.

4. Schedule or plan meals in situations that will make it difficult to purge afterward—meet a friend for lunch, go for a walk with a friend after a meal, and so on.

4. **Diet pills**—These don't work over the long run and may be toxic.

The binge and purge cycle is self-maintaining. It starts with low self-esteem and concerns about weight, and it leads to an increase in dieting, more severe dieting, loss of control, bingeing, and purging.

Dieting leads to bingeing, which leads to lowered self-esteem, heightened concerns about weight, and more dieting. Subsequent bingeing leads to purging, which again lowers self-esteem. Purging also makes people feel hungry again, which leads to more bingeing.

Because weight loss is not extreme under these circumstances, bingeing and purging can go on indefinitely. Indeed, it is a long-term and self-

If purging is such a dangerous and yet unsuccessful weight-loss technique, why do so many people persist in using it? One reason is that purging releases powerful emotions, such as anger, and gives people a sense of being in control. For another, purging can be a means of self-punishment or a way to eliminate guilt over eating. In addition, purging is powerfully reinforcing. It can protect people from weight gain and free them from restricting what they eat. Some people even get more relief from purging than they do from bingeing.

perpetuating cycle in which some people get trapped.

What bulimia feels like

Unlike people who have anroexia, people who have bulimia usaully know something is wrong. The reason for this is that people who have anorexia, and who restrict their food, can convince themselves that they are simply "being healthy" and "eating well." However, people who binge eat and then make themselves throw up cannot pretend that this is normal or healthy behavior. The symptoms don't fit into any normal pattern of eating behavior.

Almost everyone who has bulimia considers herself far too heavy or too large, and she judges her self-worth accordingly. Although she is willing to go to great lengths to make bingeing and purging a part of her life, these activities seem to intensify rather than diminish her feelings of isolation and self-deprecation.

Physical consequences

Unofficially...
You can't neces-
sarily tell that
someone has
bulimia just by
looking at him.
But the conse-
quences of hav-
ing the disorder
may be all too
apparent in
physical exams,
blood work,
and EKGs.

Although some people who have bulimia may look "healthier" than those who have anorexia, bingeing and purging create potentially serious physical problems in addition to depriving the body of nutrition. For example, during purging, acids in vomit damage the teeth, throat, esophagus, and stomach. Even more serious harm, such as stomach ruptures or heart failure, can occur during purging due to the loss of vital minerals such as sodium and potassium. When emetics are used to induce vomiting, nerve or muscle damage may result. The use of laxatives can lead to dependence, making regular bowel movements impossible. As in anorexia, bulimia may lead to irregular menstrual periods and diminished interest in sex.

The anorexia-bulimia connection

Because anorexia is associated with starvation and bulimia with gorging, they would seem to be quite different. Indeed there are significant differences, but doctors now recognize overlap points between anorexia and bulimia.

Many people who have anorexia turn to purging when restricting food no longer achieves the results they seek. Medically, it can be unclear where the boundary lies between anorexia and bulimia. For example, if a woman who has anorexia but who has begun to regain some weight and menstruate begins to binge and purge, which category does she fall into? Should she be medically placed into the category of people who have anorexia but who binge and purge, or should she be placed into the group of people who have bulimia and who purge? The distinction here is arbitrary, and most doctors aren't as concerned about categorizing people as they are about treating them. Still, the term *bulimarexia* has come into use in some circles to describe a combination of anorectic and bulimic features.

Psychological patterns

Bulimia is what psychologists call an impulse disorder. Bingeing is an impulsive act. People who have bulimia may be impulsive in other ways. They may overspend money, for example, or steal, abuse drugs or alcohol, or act out sexually. These impulses set them apart from many people who have anorexia, especially those who restrict food. At the same time, they may share some of the same impulses with people who have anorexia and who also purge.

"I am fully aware that I have bulimia. I eat too little and purge the rest, so my body lacks nutrients. Consequently, I have no energy. I am inclined to sleep an abnormal amount of time, and just going to school is exhausting for me. I am not only exhausted, but I have bad digestion and my teeth are corroding. In many places the enamel has been eaten away by stomach acids that wash over my teeth every time I throw up.

"I actually had to have one of my front teeth capped because stomach acid had eaten a hole into the back of it. My obsessive desire to be thin has completely distorted my ability to be logical and reasonable about my body. Also, I have psychological problems: My self-esteem has plummeted and I am constantly obsessing about how 'fat' I am. I always compare myself to other women and let my weight affect my moods. If I weigh 1 or 2 pounds more than my normal weight, I feel depressed and frustrated that particular day. But, if I weigh less than my normal weight, I feel elated and powerful.

"But I always keep a running tab in my head on how much more weight I need to lose. For example, when I weighed 100 pounds, I then needed to weigh 95. And when I reached that goal, I needed to weigh 90 pounds, and so on. The obsessive behavior this disorder provokes is both horrible and unrelenting. No weight loss is ever enough to make me feel as though I am 'good enough.'

"I have come to believe that my feelings of fatness are related to feelings of powerlessness. I have noticed that when I feel the fattest, my life is at the most chaotic, stressful, and out of control. And when I feel the thinnest, my life is somewhat on an even keel and under control. This wide range of emotion has left me feeling drained and tired of this sick game, yet the obsession continues."

—A young woman describing her disorder

Bulimia isn't a tougher psychological problem to treat than anorexia—both disorders are difficult to manage, but for different reasons. While people who have anorexia tend to be overly controlled, rigid, and difficult to reach psychologically, people who have bulimia tend to be more flexible, albeit more impulsive and chaotic than people who have anorexia.

Bulimia has physiological causes, perhaps including these:

- An "addiction" to extreme variations of glucose levels (blood sugar)
- The tension/relief cycle of bingeing and purging
- Changes in tryptophan levels (triggered by dieting)

At the same time, bulimia may provide victims with psychological and emotional "benefits" as well. Some of these may serve as the following "payoffs":

- A means of avoiding negative emotions, intimacy, and stress
- A form of rebellion when anger can't be expressed in a more direct way
- A last-ditch attempt to get attention for problems that are causing a great deal of pain

A possible family link

Many people who have bulimia suffer from depression or come from families that have a history of depression. Others struggle with alcohol or drug addiction. But no conclusive link exists between mood disorders or substance abuse and bulimia. In fact, some doctors have noted that many of their patients who have bulimia—and whose disordered

Watch Out!
Bulimia may be linked to low levels of the neurotransmitters seratonin and norepinephrine, both of which play a role in depression and other related psychological illnesses. A careful assessment of other disorders should be made when treatment for eating problems is being considered.

eating is only connected with a desire to control their weight and body shape—are otherwise stable.

Who has bulimia?

The people who most often have bulimia are young women. The disorder is relatively uncommon in men, although young male athletes report purging as a component of weight control. In fact, most bulimia develops as the result of a diet, even though its sufferers tend to be of average weight or some-what above average weight.

Indeed, it can be very difficult to determine when someone has bulimia. Obviously, if a person is actively purging, it's easier to tell. But what about the person who may be restricting intake, bingeing (a little), and exercising a lot? Does she have bulimia?

The best way for a professional to determine whether someone has bulimia is to find out answers to some of the following questions:

- Is the person restricting food or dieting in some other way?

- How often and to what degree does the person binge?

- Is the person engaged in some sort of activity that gets rid of ingested calories?

- Does the person feel out of control while binge-ing? (Is the activity compulsive?)

While many people may have some anorectic tendencies, such as tightly restricting their diets and perceiving their bodies through a somewhat dis-torted lens, it is harder to have a "little bit of bulimia" because this disorder involves purging, a behavior that is very hard to ignore.

> **"**
> Sometimes, say once a month or every two months, I throw up after I eat a lot. At other times I just eat very little for a day or two. My weight is average for someone my age, and I'm healthy, but I was just wondering—because I always thought an eat-ing disorder was when you did those things on a regular basis—if I have bulimia?
> —A young mother, con-cerned about her eating patterns
> **"**

In the American culture, many of us overeat on occasion and then may try to counteract it with crash diets and exercise. It's no accident that advertising and chain-store displays feature exercise machines and dieting programs right after the winter holidays, when people are most likely to overeat. But this kind of seasonal overindulgence doesn't qualify as bulimia.

As with anorexia, bulimia typically begins during adolescence. Eventually, half of the people who develop anorexia will develop bulimia. Bulimic patterns can be maintained longer than anorectic ones because the effects of starvation are slower to develop. Consequently, many people who have bulimia do not seek help until they reach their 30s or 40s.

It can be very confusing to distinguish between anorexia, bingeing/purging subtype and bulimia, nonpurging subtype. In fact, some would argue if the two are really distinct diagnoses. However, if the main emphasis is on food restriction—that person may be more in the anorectic ballpark. If the person isn't dieting strenuously, but bingeing and purging, he may be more in the bulimic spectrum. Even professionals have difficulty making precise diagnoses in this area, as the two problems are probably on a continuum.

Two views from the inside

The stories that follow illustrate bulimia's wide range of symptoms:

Lisa, who is finishing her last year of college, developed bulimia when she was 18. She regularly ate huge amounts of food but maintained her normal weight by forcing herself to vomit. Lisa often

66
I am well aware that I suffer from bulimia and have been for the past 7 years. I have decided to finally seek help because this obsession has been such a big part of my life that I couldn't stop it now even if I wanted to. In fact, I have added diet pills and alcohol to my situation.
—A young woman, concerned about the dangers of bulimia
99

felt like "an emotional powder keg"—she was angry, frightened, and depressed.

Unable to understand her own behavior, she was convinced that no one else would, either. She felt isolated and lonely. Typically, when things were not going well, she would be overcome with an uncontrollable desire for sweets. She would eat pounds of candy and cake at a time and often would not stop until she was exhausted or in severe pain. Then, overwhelmed with guilt and disgust, she would make herself vomit.

Lisa's eating habits so embarrassed her that she kept them secret until she became depressed by her mounting problems and attempted suicide. She is now in therapy and well on the way to recovery.

At 32, Jim was working as an attorney for a high-pressure corporate law firm when he began to diet and increase his hours at the gym. Anxious to be more attractive, Jim began to exercise compulsively, to the point of running 8 miles a day on the treadmill. Eventually, he removed all fat from his diet, but Jim's control finally broke down and he began to binge. He tried to vomit, but he found that he couldn't. As a consequence, Jim increased his time at the gym, exercising even on days when he was sick or in the very early hours of the morning if he had to work until quite late at night. His diagnosis: a non-vomiting form of bulimia. Exhausted and ashamed of having "a girl's disease," Jim finally sought treatment for that disorder.

Cases like those of Jim and Lisa may seem quite different and disconnected, but both illustrate low self-esteem and extreme anxiety about body image. Nevertheless, those are important links among *all* eating disorders.

Just the Facts

- Bulimia follows a self-maintaining cycle that includes both bingeing and purging.

- "Purges" can take nonvomiting forms, such as over-exercise.

- Bulimia and anorexia are different disorders, but they often have overlapping symptoms.

- Bulimia results from a combination of physiological, psychological, and environmental causes and is often triggered by dieting.

- Bulimia derives from a sense of low self-esteem.

GET THE SCOOP ON...
Binge Eating Disorder (BED) ▪ Eating
disorders: "Not Otherwise Specified"
▪ Similarities and differences between
eating disorders ▪ Warning signs ▪ Defining
"normal" eating ▪ Personal profiles

Other Eating Disorders

Given the current American preoccupation with weight, fitness, and appearance, it could be said that many of us live with *some* kind of distorted relationship with food. Of course, that is a cultural observation rather than a medical diagnosis, but it is true that professionals now recognize a far wider range of eating disorders than anorexia and bulimia. Descriptions of these disorders differ, as this chapter shows, but their sources are similar: a combination of physical, psychological, and cultural factors marked by disordered thinking about food and body image.

Binge Eating Disorder

The most common of the eating disorders after anorexia nervosa and bulimia nervosa, is Binge Eating Disorder, or BED. A relatively recent condition, BED was defined as a disorder in 1994. BED is characterized by bingeing, but the condition does not include purging.

Binge eating refers to the consumption of an unusually large quantity of food within a brief

Diagnostic Criteria for Binge Eating Disorder

Recurrent episodes of binge eating are characterized by the following:

1. Eating an amount of food that is definitely more than most people would eat in the same amount of time under similar circumstances

2. Lack of control over eating during the episode; a feeling that one cannot stop

Episodes include at least three of the following:

1. Eating more rapidly than normal

2. Eating until feeling overly full

3. Eating large amounts of food when one is not feeling physically hungry

4. Eating alone because of embarrassment over the amount one is eating

5. Feeling disgusted with oneself, depressed, guilty, or otherwise distressed after overeating

6. Episodes that occur on the average of two or more days a week for six months

period of time. The main difference between people who have bulimia and people who binge is purging: People who have bulimia follow binges with some type of purge, while people who binge-eat do not.

Although binge eating is also sometimes labeled compulsive eating, there are differences between the two. Binge eating is more often used as a clinical diagnosis, the one doctors use to define the problem. This term implies real binges—that is, large amounts of food are eaten quickly during episodes in which the person feels out of control. Compulsive overeating, on the other hand, refers to people who use food to manage stress and difficult emotions, or people who overeat rather than binge in the clinical sense. While compulsive overeating is most certainly a problem related to food, it is not an official diagnosis.

The doctors' definition

In Diagnosing Binge Eating Disorder (BED), doctors look for normal or overweight individuals who meet the criteria for bulimia nervosa but who do not practice purging. These individuals also experience feelings of loss of control and considerable distress over their eating behavior.

Sally, a freshman in college, was an athlete, and eager to maintain a slim, muscled figure. She dieted strictly, but found her control would fail, particularly at night. She started to eat her roommates' junk food in the middle of the night (since she didn't buy it herself). She would replace the food the next day, ashamed of her behavior. Her roommates began to hide their food from her. Eventually, desperate in the night, she would roam the dorm, hitting vending machines and occasionally even trash cans for binge food. She never purged, but went to bed physically full and emotionally disgusted and drained. She would wake every morning, determined to resume her dieting and "healthy" eating, and restrict food all day, only to be hungry and driven each night. After months of nighttime binges and the subsequent weight gain, she finally sought treatment.

Binge eating is not just overeating. To fit the diagnosis, a person must binge usually at least two days a week for six months. BED is not associated with other eating disorders.

The emotional aspect—self-loathing and a sense of being out of control—is also a necessary component of BED.

Who's at risk?

According to the National Institutes of Mental Health (NIMH), binge eating is a widespread affliction. Unlike anorexia and bulimia, which affect adolescent girls and young women most commonly, BED affects men and women almost equally and crosses all age and racial barriers.

As many as half of all obese people may binge eat, although only perhaps 25 percent of them fit the diagnostic criteria for BED. Binge eating is often accompanied by psychological symptoms, including depression and what psychologists call "poor impulse control" (acting out in sexual or violent ways, for example). These related conditions may create negative feedback that leads to more compulsive eating.

What's behind BED?

Binge eating may be a response to repeated efforts at dieting because deprivation of certain foods may create cravings, which then lead to gorging. As with other eating disorders, this dieting is tied to a distorted perception of what one's body should look like.

Other psychological factors include using food as a form of relief from negative feelings and a need to isolate oneself from people because of the unconscious theory that "nobody likes a fat person." The

Bright Idea
People who seem to be constantly struggling with an overweight problem should have a professional assessment for eating disorders. Binge eating can be treated, with results that are more effective than going on another diet.

Warning Signs of Binge Eating Disorder (BED)

- Frequent, repeated eating, either as secretive bouts or as constant snacking

- A sense of being out of control, with an apparent inability to stop

- Feelings of shame and self-disgust

- Overweight appearance

- Depression

- History of diet failures

Source: Anorexia Nervosa and Related Eating Disorders, Inc. (ANRED), a nonprofit clearinghouse that distributes information about anorexia nervosa, bulimia, Binge Eating Disorder (BED) and other less well-known eating disorders. All information is free and available on the World Wide Web at http:// www.anred.com. The site is revised and updated monthly. (Please see Appendix B for further information on resources such as ANRED.)

---

resulting feelings of loneliness stimulate more self-punishing eating.

While a person may not be able to see these connections for herself, she probably does know that something is wrong with her behavior, and she may feel intense shame about it.

Physical consequences of bingeing

Many of the physical ill effects of binge eating match those of obesity because both involve excessive eating. But the pace of bingeing, combined with the kinds of foods most often chosen by people who binge-eat—sweets and other carbohydrates—magnify the ill effects. Hazards include high blood pressure, high cholesterol levels, hardening of the arteries, heart disease, strokes, and heart attacks. Overindulgence in sweets and junk food places

Unofficially...
Binge eating disorder is self-perpetuating. The inability to stop overeating helps feed the guilt, anxiety, and depression that keeps the compulsive cycle of this disorder going.

stress on the pancreas and lowers glucose levels in the blood, which can eventually result in diabetes.

In fact, the American Diabetes Association has expressed a particular interest in BED and is now a resource for information and treatment. As more attention is given to eating disorders, there is heightened realization of the long-term health effects.

E.D.—Not Otherwise Specified

Because most people who have an eating disorder don't meet the full criteria for a diagnosis of anorexia, bulimia, or BED, a new term has been coined: "Eating Disorder, Not Otherwise Specified" (ED-NOS).

Who has an ED-NOS?

Defining a term as general as "not otherwise specified" may seem tricky, but doctors use this label for a variety of eating disorders. For example, "Eating Disorder, Not Otherwise Specified" might refer to a woman who has anorexia but who still menstruates, or whose weight is still normal. ED-NOS may identify someone who purges without bingeing—who induces vomiting, for instance, after eating only a small quantity of food. The term might describe a combination of anorectic and bulimic features that includes starvation as well as bingeing and purging. Or, it might describe someone who binges and purges only on occasion. These variations on more clearly categorized eating disorders don't fit the textbook definitions, but they definitely qualify as some kind of disorder.

Likewise, an ED-NOS may refer to periodic binge eating that goes beyond the occasional overeating in which most people indulge.

Or, the term may be applied to any kind of unhealthy eating pattern that is accompanied by disordered body perceptions or overreactive emotions, whether it fits a standard definition or not. In these instances, people are doing more than simply taking in too much or too little food; clearly they are in some kind of psychological pain and are in danger of hurting themselves physically.

Compulsive overeating

As noted earlier, compulsive overeating isn't an official diagnosis of an eating disorder. The term is most often used to describe emotional overeating. However, some experts make a clearer distinction between compulsive overeating and BED. For example, compulsive overeaters are characterized as having an addiction to food, using food and eating as a way to hide from their emotions, to fill a void they feel inside, and to cope with daily stresses and problems in their lives.

Compulsive overeaters tend to be overweight and are usually aware that their eating habits are abnormal. Their distress is intensified by cultural stereotyping of "fat people." Dieting is almost as painful to a compulsive overeater as eating is to someone with anorexia. The health consequences of obesity, which may result from this pattern of

Watch Out!
Some people make a practice of chewing but not swallowing. They simply spit out whatever food they have put in their mouths. The behavior is not as noticeable as others might be, but it may be just as hazardous because it denies the body the nutrients it needs.

66

I began to use food to suppress my emotions. I wasn't going to use drugs and alcohol anymore, but I still had all these issues that were unresolved. I needed something with which to medicate myself.
—A young woman who began a food addiction after she stopped using drugs and alcohol

99

David, a man in his mid-40s, has diabetes, which he can't control because he can't control his eating. For David, compulsive overeating and obesity have had serious consequences: His diabetes has worsened and has affected his eyes and feet. David has had heart surgery as well, but despite the serious condition of his health, he feels compelled to eat *all* of whatever it is he happens to be eating.

compulsive overeating, include risks for a heart attack, high blood pressure and cholesterol, kidney disease and/or failure, arthritis and bone deterioration, and stroke.

Night eating and other disordered eating patterns

Some less well-known eating problems may not affect large numbers of people, nor are they recognized by specialists as official disorders. Nonetheless, they represent *eating patterns* that can be very disturbing to the people who suffer from them. Night eating, for example, is more of a symptom of a problem than a disorder in itself. As a pattern of behavior, it applies to many people who have other eating problems, such as bulimia and BED.

Nocturnal Sleep-Related Eating

This disordered pattern of behavior consists of recurring bouts of sleepwalking, during which a person binges on large quantities of foods that are unusually sugary or fatty. Most often, sufferers do not remember these episodes. However, this seemingly unconscious eating pattern poses the same health risks as other forms of compulsive overeating (in addition to the dangers of sleepwalking).

People who suffer from Nocturnal Sleep-Related Eating tend to be overweight, and it's thought that their problem is connected to various dieting attempts.

Night Eating Syndrome

Likewise, Night Eating Syndrome is connected to weight-reduction diets and irregular eating patterns. The people who suffer from it put off eating any food at all until the evening, when they binge eat. Consequently, they have trouble falling asleep or staying asleep. This pattern is sometimes seen among people who have disorders such as bulimia.

Unofficially...
Pica, a widely misunderstood phenomenon, is defined as a compulsive craving for non-food items, such as dirt, sand, clay, paste, and ice, or foods that contain no nutrition. Pica is not considered an eating disorder per se, but it is a peculiar pattern that is present almost exclusively in children.

Prader-Willi syndrome is another dysfunctional eating pattern marked by an insatiable appetite. It's not an eating disorder in the usual sense and is quite rare, but it should be considered if a child, in particular, develops an excessive appetite.

In addition, both Nocturnal Sleep-Related Eating and Night Eating Syndrome are associated with stress and fatigue. This is understandable, given enough sleep deprivation, but stress may also result from frustrating efforts to match externally imposed body standards. If one is obsessively concerned with, say, looking as skinny as the models in glossy magazines, or as muscular as the *Baywatch* jocks, it can twist one's entire approach to life by creating an unceasing inner tension.

Common threads

Whether night eating or pica, overeating or self-starvation, these separate conditions share a few common themes and elements. For example, virtually everyone who sufferers from these conditions also suffers from low self-esteem.

The prime motivator for most people who suffer from an eating disorder is a conscious or unconscious need for control. In an unmanageable world, the one thing these people can always control is diet. When eating gets out of control, they can react by purging, limiting, or obsessing over only a few particular foods to get a sense of control over their life.

All eating disorders are hazardous to our health: They endanger the arteries, bones, vital organs, and even the brain, depending on the disease. All have emotional pain in common, both as cause and effect. One group of people who are susceptible to developing eating disorders are people who have diabetes.

The diabetes connection

The body's ability to properly manage glucose levels (blood sugar) is thrown off by both diabetes and eating disorders. More research is needed to link

> **"**
> I just wish I knew what was going on inside my head when I became bulimic again. It seems weird and ironic that in order for me to gain some sense of control in my life, I have to engage in something that makes me feel as though I have no control.
> —A young woman who relapsed during her recovery from bulimia
> **"**

these elements, but there are obvious connections. For example, diabetes requires an almost obsessive focus on food that can easily evolve into the rigidly controlled behaviors of an eating disorder—including the view that some foods are "dangerous."

No one questions care in eating or even weight loss in someone who has diabetes, so an eating disorder can stay hidden even longer than it might in other circumstances. Given the potential links, the Diabetes Association is a good source of information and advice on eating disorders.

Unofficially...
Whatever the eating disorder, the experts say that the key to getting free of the cycle is to eliminate dieting.

So what *is* a normal eating pattern?

Because so many of us have difficulties with food and weight—not to mention feelings of inadequacy about our bodies and how much we weigh—many of our eating habits could be labeled "disordered." Absurd as that may sound, it's important to have a clearer picture of what "normal" is if we are to gain any understanding of what eating disorders really are.

You may be surprised to learn that the losing battle so many people wage with the scale might actually be the result of unrealistic weight expectations instead of a sign of inadequacy, failure, or loss of control. In the pursuit of a slim body that measures up to rigid cultural expectations, many men and women unwittingly establish anorectic patterns.

The good news is that there are effective treatments as well as professional programs that can help in setting realistic weight goals and improving self-image.

Most people who have eating disorders do not fit into the precise, clinical diagnoses of a particular disorder. In other words, a person who has anorexia may not have a skeletal appearance (as we might expect), despite rigid food restrictions. A person who has bulimia may not vomit after every meal, but

Sally was a somewhat chubby baby who was put on a diet as an infant and given only skim milk to drink. The constant attention paid to her weight during childhood drove her underground: Sally baked her own cakes and cookies and collected bottles for change so that she could buy sweets after school because her mother didn't keep "fattening foods" in the house.

A "successful" diet in fifth grade caused Sally to lose a lot of weight and taught her that much of what she was eating was "bad" for her. She has been on a series of diets ever since. Although her weight has never been far above normal, her everyday life has involved a pattern of overeating, dieting, and feeling bad about herself. She was well into middle age before another malady sent her into treatment, which, as a side effect, helped her become aware of the self-destructive nature of her attitudes. Once Sally began to accept herself in other ways, she could take the focus off her weight, which eventually came into a healthy balance.

> 66
> There is no size you are supposed to be. What's important is not your size or the amount of weight you've gained or lost, but the quality of the life you lead. Does the size of our bodies indicate the size of our lives? Success comes from living, not from waiting for some magical moment when all of the requirements you have placed on yourself have been met. It's not the size of your body that counts, it's the size of your life.
> —A young woman in recovery from a serious eating disorder
> 99

she might overexercise to compensate for perceived overeating. Someone who binge-eats may not consume tens of thousands of calories in a few hours, but he might feel compelled to overeat, even while realizing that the behavior is irrational.

Under the media barrage of model-thin bodies, it's hard to find the line between a typical misperception of one's image and a pathological one. For example, a size-12 woman may not like how she looks in a bathing suit because she compares herself unfavorably with the size 2 model who advertises the same suit. The difference between this woman and the young girl who wears a size 4 but sees herself as obese is really only a matter of degree.

"Normal" people don't actually spend much time or energy thinking about their food intake. But given the context of a culture obsessed with being thin, very few of us are not thoroughly educated in reading labels and eating healthy within the limits of whatever eating trend happens to be in vogue.

Many people who "eat healthy" do so to improve their diet. So how are you expected to know when this kind of attention to what you eat becomes disordered? Most experts agree that it is best to err on the safe side if you have any doubts at all:—Because these conditions tend to be progressive, it's a good idea to get an evaluation as soon as possible from a professional who is trained in determining what is "normal."

Familiar stories

The following stories illustrate patterns of disordered eating that might seem familiar to you, given that so many of us share at least some aspects of these eating patterns.

Many of us turn to "comfort foods" when we are stressed or exhausted. Whether it's a cheeseburger and fries, a baked potato, or Mom's rice pudding, there *are* tough times when most people crave a little something to make them feel safe and cozy. Compare that with the compulsive overeater, who says: "I used to use food to take the edge off life. I tried to control my food, but I couldn't. I hated my body, so in turn I hated myself. If only I could lose weight and eat like normal people, I thought, then I would be okay."

People who aren't compulsive about food don't connect "weight" and "hate" or think about what "normal" people eat. Nor do they feel guilty about having an extra snack on occasion.

Likewise, most of us splurge occasionally on special meals during the holidays or at a restaurant, even when we are on our own. And most of us keep a few treats around the house for when we feel like having one. That's different from the person who says of her eating:

> "I could not have a loaf of bread in the house because I would have to eat it all, one slice after another until it was gone and I was miserable. I used to order Chinese food for six people and then eat it all myself. I would tell myself that I had ordered so much food in order to have leftovers. There was never anything left over, of course, except the feeling of being so full and so full of self-disgust."

Then there are all of us who go on diets to lose a little of the "extra" weight we put on over the holidays, or to get ready for bathing-suit season. This dieting pattern (which may or may not succeed) is a far cry from this perpetual dieter's experience:

> "I would go to diet clubs to lose some weight, but then I'd lose control. I gained 100 pounds in a few years, which I lost and gained again in increments as the years went on. This crazy cycle of controlled eating and then bingeing ran my life for over 20 years."

The line between "normal" eating and disordered eating may be a fine one, but those who have gone over that line even a bit may be living lives of self-torture.

Just the Facts

- Eating disorders that have differing symptoms often stem from similar causes.

- Most eating disorders can be successfully treated once they are recognized.

- A need for "control" is the psychological connector among eating disorders.

- Paying attention to eating for good health does not necessarily cross the line into eating-related obsessions.

GET THE SCOOP ON...
The line between enough and too much
■ The connection between eating disorders
and exercise ■ Athletes and disordered
eating ■ Personal profiles

Exercise Disorders

"Fitness" is almost as much a part of the American psyche as "diet"—and it's almost as easy to abuse. Many athletes, for example, develop eating disorders as a result of their training, while some people who already have an eating disorder use overexercise as a form of purging. Still others whose disordered thinking focuses primarily on exercise rather than food use it as a tool for weight control. Yet in the American culture, an excessive focus on the body is rarely viewed as a problem.

Just as many of us have been raised to believe that dieting is "normal," some people are even more convinced that exercise is good. Today fitness is a multibillion-dollar industry, with tens of thousands of health clubs across the nation filled to capacity with people who squeeze hours of exercise into already packed schedules.

What does it say about modern American society that virtually every infomercial—paid programming on TV—is a high-pressure sales pitch for food, diet, or exercise equipment? Channel-surfers can flit from the food network to almost daylong offerings of exercise programs and dieting advice. It's no wonder that attitudes toward eating and exercise get confused.

Exercise is *good,* isn't it?

Yes, exercise is beneficial. Health experts suggest that if people expended more energy through moderate exercise, they wouldn't need to waste so much time with diets.

Exercise assets

There's also no question that the benefits of exercise are many. Physical activity is relaxing, stress-reducing, and invigorating. Exercise improves the strength and tone of a variety of muscles, not only so that we move with more comfort, but also so that our organs function more effectively. Regular aerobic exercise increases the effectiveness of the heart and cardiovascular system, which maintains the entire body. All these benefits derive from the expenditure of 2,000 to 3,500 calories each week through activities such as running, jogging, dancing, brisk walking, and the like.

Good health benefits can be attained through 30 minutes of exercise a day for six days a week, or through less strenuous efforts such as gardening or playing golf for an hour a day five days a week. Building and maintaining muscle and bone mass require weight-bearing exercise, however, which varies according to age and level of fitness. But simply carrying light weights on a 30-minute walk three times a week may be sufficient to keep bones and muscles healthy.

Exercise liabilities

Although the health benefits of moderate, regular exercise are undeniable, too much exercise can be hazardous. After 3,500 hundred calories are burned per week, health benefits actually decrease, and the risk of injury increases. Overdoing weight-bearing exercise can tear or break down muscle tissue instead of building it, and it can damage bones, joints, cartilage, tendons, and ligaments.

Apart from the physical downside of too much exercise are the negative psychological consequences as well, when exercise becomes the primary focus of life and pushes all other interests aside.

When exercise becomes too much of a good thing

Exercise abuse, also called obligatory exercising or anorexia athletica, creates even more physical, mental, and emotional damage than the anxiety generated by overcompetitiveness. When self-worth is based only on physique and sports performance, and when relationships are abandoned in favor of aerobics, then overexercise has become a problem. Even worse, when a person who overexercises abuses steroids and related drugs, the danger and potential for disaster multiply.

Still, it's often difficult to recognize when there's a problem: Exercise seems like such a healthy outlet for energy.

Unlike anorexia, bulimia, and Binge Eating Disorder, compulsive exercising is not a clinical diagnosis in itself—but it may be a symptom of an eating disorder. Many people who are preoccupied with food and weight exercise compulsively as a method of controlling their weight. Even when food is not involved, compulsive exercise is connected to the patterns of disordered eating because the real issues are not weight and performance excellence; the problems revolve around power, control, and self-mastery.

Moneysaver
There's no need to spend a small fortune on gym fees and exercise equipment when you can maintain fitness at no cost through such activities as brisk walking or simple gardening.

An unhealthy relationship

Overexercise has been linked with disordered eating and negative body perception in a variety of ways. As previously noted, compulsive exercise can in itself be a means of purging, but there are more subtle connections.

Regular exercise programs or competitive sports can increase dissatisfaction with body image and encourage dieting, especially among young women whose self-esteem may be shaky. The focus on physical appearance that is naturally fostered by gyms and spas adds to the level of anxiety and image distortion experienced by those who are prone to eating disorders.

Overexercise is very often viewed as a warning sign by professionals who diagnose eating disorders because exercise is one of the means used to purge or counteract calorie intake.

Warning Signs of Overexercise

These are some of the warning signs that a person may be exercising too much. Does that person:

- Engage in repeated physical activities that far exceed requirements for good health?

- Exercise rather than work or socialize?

- Focus on exercise as work rather than fun?

- Keep challenging herself, despite her achievements and without enjoying them?

- Define self-worth in terms of athletic achievements but is never satisfied?

- Keep detailed performance records and constantly focus on perfection?

- Justify excesses by saying he's "special"?

Is it an addiction?

Overexercise is labeled compulsive when a person feels compelled to exercise, or obligatory when a person feels obliged to exercise. One theory is that addiction develops as a result of certain brain chemicals that are released into the body during vigorous exercise.

Whether or not this theory proves to be true, athletes do talk about a "runner's high." But exercise addicts not only feel euphoria following vigorous sessions—they also experience guilt and anxiety and even go through a form of withdrawal when they are unable to exercise.

Over the line

American society values and seems to demand slim, well-toned, agile, and beautiful bodies for both men and women of all ages. Although this preoccupation with appearance may have grown out of a concern for health, the results—unreasonable expectations and physical demands—are less healthy. Some people these days may not be satisfied with their bodies, but obligatory exercisers take their dissatisfaction even further. They are completely focused on their sport or their training schedule; when they're injured, they work out anyway.

As with compulsive dieting, compulsive exercise is part of an effort to enhance self-esteem, meet emotional needs, and hide from emotional pain. Overexercisers keep increasing their efforts, hoping that it will eventually solve all their problems—of course, it won't.

66

I pay careful attention to trainers who spend too much of their free time at work and begin to look a bit too sinewy. We want healthy exercise, not excess.—Laura, a health club manager

99

The connection with eating disorders

Exercise is used to excess by people with bulimia as a way to purge, and by people with anorexia as a nonpurging way to control weight. There's also a

Timesaver
Five hours a week, tops, is all the exercise that's really needed. Why spend more time than that?

theory that in some cases excessive physical activity actually causes anorexia. Researchers have found that laboratory rats whose food is regulated will exercise more and eat even less, until eventually they die of starvation. The same pattern can be observed in some overexercisers who resent taking time out to eat.

For the compulsive exerciser, the surface goal may be to burn calories, just as it is for most people with eating disorders. The ultimate reward, however, is a sense of temporary power, control, or self-respect, whether achieved through excessive exercise or through extreme restraints on eating.

The non-athlete who is recovering from an eating disorder may face an increased risk of developing some form of compulsive exercise behavior. It's easy to convince one's self that exercise is taking care of the body and that it's not really purging after all. This attitude can quickly lead to compulsive exercise as a replacement for food restriction or

---

A college student who has always struggled to satisfy her need to be perfect added athletics to her quest for both perfect grades and extracurricular stardom. During her junior year, under pressure from the demands of team soccer, track, and the school play, she began to feel that her life was out of control. She decided that if she was perfect on the outside, she would feel better on the inside. She began to exercise all the time: She ran 5 to 6 miles every day and did 400 sit-ups every night when she came home. Even though she ran with plastic wrap taped around her body, she still couldn't "sweat away" enough fat from her thighs to feel "perfect."

purging. Doctors supervise exercise as carefully as they supervise diet in patients who have eating disorders.

Who overdoes it?

In addition to people who have—or who are susceptible to—eating disorders, there are others who are encouraged to overexercise, sometimes from a very early age. For example, parents feel safe encouraging their kids to exercise: It keeps them out of trouble, burns off excess energy, and gives them lots of fresh air.

But exercise can become problematic when kids and young people focus on athletics as a way of pleasing their parents. Because competitive sports are being introduced at increasingly younger ages—toddler soccer, junior football, and the like—athletics have become an easy and socially acceptable way to get Mom or Dad's attention and approval. All too often parental praise for athletic skill can evolve into an almost exclusive appreciation for children's physical selves and the assumption that "good bodies" mean "good people."

Eating disorders in athletes

The emphasis on physical appearance increases with age because of the value and importance society places on youth, fitness, and success. For many athletes, competitive pressures are satisfied by compulsive dieting, at least for a while.

To make things even more complicated, not all weight and body image fears are expressed through food. Exercise is a tool, too. These days obsessive exercising seems to affect an even wider age range of people than most eating disorders. Trying to run off middle-age spread can become an obsession—and daily games of handball can make even the

"
I began to exercise twice a day, running in the afternoon alone and later in my room at night with my roommate. We would run barefoot in our underwear in front of a mirror so that we could see how our bodies looked. I was sore all the time. My knees and hips ached, but I liked it. I enjoyed the pain. It seemed normal. I felt athletic.
—A college student who became obsessed with her weight
"

Unofficially...
Athletes who participate in sports such as gymnastics, figure skating, dancing, and synchronized swimming have a higher percentage of eating disorders than those who ski or play basketball or volleyball. In the early 1990s, the American College of Sports Medicine reported that 62 percent of female athletes in sports such as figure skating and gymnastics were affected by eating disorders.

grayest 47-year-old feel like a youth again. Undoubtedly, you've seen the personification of the classic "anorectic female" at the gym—a woman who always seems to be there, no matter what time you happen to go. An emaciated woman with an intense expression, she spends 30 minutes or more on each piece of aerobic equipment and then does hundreds of abdominal exercises.

While many athletes resort to overdieting and overexercising to please a favorite coach or win an important match, dancers, runners, gymnasts, figure skaters and wrestlers seem to be prone to disordered eating in particular. This is especially true right before a match or performance, when weight limits are enforced, or if the sport places an overemphasis on extreme slenderness. The horrible irony in these cases is that dieting and exercising to excess makes them more vulnerable to serious injury.

Athletes who have eating disorders may also be at a higher risk for medical complications, such as an electrolyte imbalance that might lead to heart problems. Strenuous physical activity puts a lot of pressure on the body, and having an eating disorder puts the body at an even greater risk for cardiac arrest.

Different risks for male and female athletes

The National Collegiate Athletic Association reports that female athletes are doubly at risk for the development of an eating disorder. This is because they face constant social pressure to be thin and also must measure up to the demands of a sports culture that overvalues performance and low body fat and that idealizes unrealistic body shapes and sizes. Women who become sports celebrities are especially vulnerable to eating disorders.

Are You Becoming a Compulsive or Addictive Exerciser?

1. How many days or hours do you exercise per week? Do you allow time for your body to rest and recuperate?

2. How rigid are you about your exercise schedule? Can you skip days or sessions without anxiety?

3. Do you force yourself to exercise when you're sick or tired?

4. If you're an outdoors exerciser, are you out in all kinds of weather?

5. If the weather keeps you inside, do you have to "make it up" in some way?

6. Do you go out of your way to schedule exercise? For example, do you go to the gym after midnight or get up at 3:00 in the morning to run or work out?

If you answered "yes" to more than three of these questions and "no" to the first two, you might want to check in with an eating disorders specialist.

Bright Idea
Give your own routine a checkup. Experts point to two key warning signs of exercise addiction:

1. Is your sport or workout schedule fun? If it is, you're still okay.

2. If you can back off from exercising when your doctor or family expresses concern that you are hurting yourself or losing perspective, you are within the safety zone.

Men also develop eating disorders, but not to the extent that women do. This is partly because their bodies naturally carry less fat than women. Their metabolisms are faster as well, so weight is easier to control.

Many successful women athletes boast of bodies that are as lean, muscular, and sinewy as a man's. However, actually attaining this physique can cost

Watch Out!
It's not only pro athletes who are at risk of developing eating and exercise disorders. School and college competitors who overdiet while trying to compete also put themselves at risk for collapse and even death. What's more, they tend not to win because they haven't eaten enough to fuel themselves!

women their "femaleness" when they stop menstruating and lose the capacity to bear children. Alterations in body chemistry and overexercise, which presumably enhance women's strength, often result in the brittle bones of osteoporosis.

The inside scoop

There is nothing "typical" about anyone who suffers from exercise addiction. The disorder cuts a wide swath across society:

A young woman, Maria, had bulimia for six years and used exercise to control her weight. She says of her addiction: "I was wasting away. I had no energy in my legs anymore. I was exercising compulsively, and routinely added 40 minutes on an exercise bike after each two-hour workout."

Then there's George, a 30-year-old man who has anorexia. After he broke his leg, George was forced to rest in bed and to limit physical activity for weeks. Instead, he ignored his doctor's advice and went out walking for hours, despite the pain, because his anxiety about not exercising was so difficult to ignore.

Or consider Ted, a man who has bulimia but who doesn't purge. Ted had a high-powered job where he often worked until 1:00 or 2:00 in the morning. Afterward, he'd spend two hours in the gym before going home.

Moderation in exercise is the best recommendation for good health, just as it is with the consumption of food. However, obsessive exercise is probably easier to conceal than other disordered patterns—which gives us all the more reason to know the danger signs.

Just the Facts

- Overexercise can be just as obsessively dangerous as overdieting.

- Exercise may be a cause as well as a result of an eating disorder.

- Compulsive exercise disorder is common among athletes, but it does not exclude many other groups of people.

- Treatment for exercise compulsion is similar to what is used for people who have food obsessions.

Responding to Danger Signals

GET THE SCOOP ON...
Why clues can be hard to see ▪ Who's at
risk? ▪ Keys to each disorder ▪ Where
the line gets crossed

PART III

Chapter 8

How to Read the Telltale Signs

Every eating disorder has a specific set of symptoms by which it is diagnosed (as described in Part II: "Eating Disorders"). One might assume that in their extreme forms, some of these disorders should be fairly easy to notice: a skeletal-looking body, obvious signs of vomiting and diarrhea, hours spent each day at the gym, and so on. But many eating disorders don't reach these dramatic stages. They are less visible and have fewer telltale signs.

Why clues are hidden

A very important common characteristic of people who have eating disorders is that they keep their condition hidden from other people. Even those nearest to the victim may participate in this deceit unconsciously, through a mechanism that is common to all eating disorders: denial.

Watch Out!
Here's another
example of
denial: A woman
in her 40s who
has had bulimia
since adoles-
cence has lost
her teeth and
hair. Neither she
nor her parents
think she has a
problem.

The power of denial

Denial is more than a refusal to admit that something might be wrong: It's a deep-seated psychological inability to see a problem.

Denial may be difficult to understand for anyone
who has never been in a situation he didn't want to
see. And it may be equally hard to believe that under
certain circumstances evidence simply can't be seen,
even if it is placed directly in front of you. Nonetheless, denial is a psychological fact—and a very
understandable one.

Some families are so frightened of what an eating disorder might mean that they don't allow
themselves to admit that there's a problem. Or, relationships within a family may be so confused and
conflicted that it seems safer to ignore a serious situation rather than endanger family stability. Young
people who have eating disorders sometimes adopt
a rebellious, antisocial mode. Their overtly self-
destructive behavior, bad attitudes, petty crimes, and
disruptions at school cause so much concern—and
create such an effective screen—that parents and
other adults may not be able to see signs of disordered eating.

On the other hand, many people who have eating disorders seem to be in complete control of
their lives. This makes it difficult for the parents of
a 15-year-old child who is tidy, good-mannered,
active in extracurricular activities, and a straight-A
student to admit there's a problem.

Denial becomes doubly powerful when the victim herself is honestly unable to see that there's a
problem. In fact, denial is the most hazardous threat
to the life and well-being of someone who has an
eating disorder because it delays treatment.

Here's an example of how difficult it is to identify an eating disorder if only a few symptoms are apparent:

A young woman was dumped by her boyfriend of six months. Following the break-up, she lost 10 pounds, which she explained was the result of depression and loss of appetite. (Weight loss is very common in depression and is often simply a stress response that has nothing to do with eating problems.) However, careful professional questioning about how she viewed her body revealed her intense concerns about feeling unattractive and distress over her weight and the appearance of her body. She admitted that although she was truly depressed, she was deliberately restricting her intake of food to lose weight and feel better about herself.

Did this young woman meet the full criteria for anorexia?

No, but she had a number of symptoms that, if not addressed, could have developed into a full-fledged eating disorder.

The culture of food control

Sometimes the inability to recognize an eating disorder derives from a force more subtle than denial. People who have lived with even mildly disordered thinking about food or body image—in themselves or in others—may not be aware that anything is out of the ordinary. They may assume that everybody lives the way they do, and their way of life is so fully reinforced by the surrounding culture that an eating disorder may not seem possible.

If "everybody" is on a diet, then dieting does not seem like such a pathological activity. If everyone's

Bright Idea
If you suspect that someone you know has an eating disorder and you want to help, look for clues: You can use signs of vomiting or laxative wrappers or diuretic packages found in the trash to confront him with reality.

"ideal" is to be underweight, then being "too skinny" doesn't seem out of the ordinary.

Tricky symptoms

Timesaver
When observing signs such as weight loss or obsessive exercise in someone who is susceptible to eating disorders, don't just worry and wonder. Gather as much information as you can about the problem, and then share it with the person.

Even professionals in the field know that it can be difficult to diagnose an eating disorder accurately, especially when symptoms are not clear-cut or if a person doesn't have all the symptoms of a given disorder.

Yet diagnosing an eating disorder *early* offers more hope for recovery than catching it after it has had time to progress to a more serious level. So whether you are a sufferer or an observer, it is important to be aware of the signs that indicate more than a suspicion of an eating disorder.

Who's at risk?

While it is now accepted that there is no typical profile of someone who has an eating disorder, the most visible symptoms might include these:

- An unnecessary focus on food, weight, and diet
- Extreme behavior related to food and exercise

Either of these should trigger a warning signal that you or someone you know might have an eating disorder.

Personal characteristics

So far, some of the most commonly observed characteristics of a person who has an eating disorder have been identified as these:

- Anger or absence of anger
- A conflicted family or a perfectionist family
- Body-image distortions
- Low self-worth
- Pessimism
- Depression

- Poor relationships

- Anxiety

- Loneliness

- Insecurity

- An obsession with the possibility of gaining weight

The likelihood that there is an eating disorder multiplies with the number of symptoms that apply.

The most likely candidates for an eating disorder are young white women, but as previous chapters have shown, these are not the only people who are susceptible to eating disorders. If the habits, behaviors, or attitudes about food surface in someone you know of any age, sex, or race, it's worth taking a closer look. Here are several specific characteristics to look for:

1. Preoccupation with details, rules, lists, order, organization, or schedules

2. Extreme perfectionism

3. Excessive devotion to work and productivity to the exclusion of leisure activities and friendships

4. Overconscientiousness, scrupulosity, and inflexibility about matters of morality, ethics, or values

5. Inability to discard worn-out or worthless objects even when they have no sentimental value

6. Reluctance to delegate tasks or to work with others unless they submit exactly to her way of doing things

7. A miserly spending style (toward himself and others)

8. Rigidity and stubbornness

Unofficially...
It may be difficult to recognize when someone has an eating disorder because hiding it is so important to the person who has one. In fact, deception is an essential component of these disorders. The outward appearance of someone who has an eating disorder does *not* always reveal the degree of physical danger that person may be in or the emotional conflicts that might be tearing her apart.

Also watch out for the following background signals:

- **Deception.** Lying about food intake and sneaking food. Lying to avoid eating and hiding the use of laxatives, diuretics, and purging.

- **Depression.** Mood swings, lack of motivation, feelings of hopelessness, anxiety or panic attacks, claustrophobia, isolation, and loneliness. Depression often accompanies eating disorders, and regardless of whether it is the cause or the effect, it *can* lead to suicide.

Family background

It can be very insightful to look into the family background of someone whom you suspect of having an eating disorder. The stereotypical family is overly demanding and rigid, but other family environments can foster eating disorders as well. In families that don't pay enough attention to their children, eating problems sometimes become a means to get the attention children crave. On the other hand, families that are smothering and that pay too much attention to the children's every move may drive the children to eating disorders as a means of escape. Dysfunctional and disorderly families very often become a matrix for eating disorders among children who manipulate food as a way of gaining more control in general.

Again, no one set of family clues can confirm suspicions of an eating disorder. However, sometimes they coexist with other telling behaviors in a family, such as the presence of alcoholism, drug addiction, or other unhealthy compulsions. Putting together the whole picture may confirm that an individual's eating habits are not just odd.

Table 8.1 reviews the telltale signs of eating disorders, their diagnoses, their symptoms, and their behavior patterns. If you see any disordered behavior or attitudes that seem familiar or that apply either to yourself or someone you know, take notice. Also note that a person does not need to display even close to all the symptoms to be suffering from a disorder.

Clues to pay attention to

Lots of other clues might point to an eating disorder as well. For example, complaints about any of the following discomforts could signal a serious health problem. Be aware that complaints such as these may be easy to ignore because they are not directly related to eating.

Anorexia or Bulimia:

- Frequent headaches due to lowered blood pressure and decreased oxygen supply to the brain.

- Coldness caused by a loss of the insulating layer of fat and/or decreased circulation due to lowered blood pressure, slowed heart rate, and slowed metabolism.

- Irregular and/or slow heart rate. Low blood pressure caused by low potassium in the blood.

- Electrolyte imbalances and vitamin deficiencies.

- Tingling in the hands, feet, and face. Vitamin deficiency, specifically potassium. Electrolyte imbalances and malnutrition. Victims often tire easily and feel light-headed.

- Dizziness, lightheadedness, and faint feeling. Caused by purging and/or laxative abuse, slowed heart rate, malnutrition and dehydration, and depression and/or stress.

TABLE 8.1 KEYS TO THE DISORDERS

Disorder	Diagnosis	Physical Symptoms	Behavior to Watch
Anorexia Nervosa	Loss of weight to 15% below normal. Absence of menstruation 3 months or delayed start of menses. Refusal to maintain weight. Intense fear of gaining weight.	Dry skin, brittle hair, and hair loss. Malnutrition and hormonal imbalances. Growth of fine hair (lanugo) on face, back, and arms. A drawn, underweight body that feels cold even in warm weather or in warm rooms. Electrolyte imbalances, vitamin deficiencies (specifically potassium), and malnutrition. Tingling in hands, feet, face. Fatigue, dizziness, lightheadedness, feeling faint—caused by malnutrition, purging and/or laxative abuse; dehydration, slowed heart rate, depression, and/or stress.	Will not eat enough due to fear of becoming fat. Eats tiny amount of low-fat, low-calorie food. Overexercises to lose weight and stay thin. May also vomit or use other forms of purging.
Bulimia Nervosa	Recurrent episodes of binge eating ("binge" meaning eating an unusually large amount of food in less time than one might normally, and having a sense of no control over eating during the episode). Recurrent inappropriate compensatory behavior to prevent weight gain, such as self-induced vomiting; misuse of laxatives, diuretics, enemas, or other medications; fasting; or excessive exercising. Episodes occur at least twice a week for 3 months.	Bruised or callused knuckles and fingers from sticking fingers in mouth and down throat to induce vomiting. Sore throat and/or swollen glands from irritation caused by stomach acids during purging. Electrolyte imbalances, vitamin deficiencies (specifically potassium), and malnutrition. Tingling in hands, feet, face. Fatigue, dizziness, lightheadedness, feeling faint—caused by malnutrition, purging and/or laxative abuse, dehydration, slowed heart rate, depression, and /or stress.	Eats unusually large amounts of food in short time periods. Binges and might purge. Purging may involve vomiting, fasting; use of laxatives, diet pills, diuretics or over-exercise. Fears "fatness." Prone to mood swings. Takes lengthy visits to bathroom after meals. Purchases large amounts of food that suddenly disappears. Laxative or diuretic wrappers appear in the trash after an unexplained disappearance of food. Has unusual swelling around the jaw. May have money problems due to the huge amount of money spent on groceries.

Disorder	Diagnosis	Physical Symptoms	Behavior to Watch
Binge Eating Disorder (BED)	Normal or overweight individuals who meet the criteria for bulimia nervosa, but who do not practice purging. Experiences feelings of loss of control and considerable distress over eating behavior. Recurrent episodes of binge eating are characterized by: Eating an amount of food that is definitely more than most people would eat in the same amount of time under similar circumstances. Lack of control over eating during the episode.	Tendency to be warm or hot, exhausted, dizzy, due to increased exertion placed on body by excess weight and increased digestive activities. Decreased endurance. Fast and/or irregular heart rate. High blood pressure caused by increased weight gain and possible raised cholesterol levels. Joint pain caused by additional stresses on the body brought on by excess weight. Fatigue. Poor circulation due to constricted veins and arteries. Varicose and spider veins. Muscle soreness, decreased mobility. Nutritional and hormonal imbalances.	Eats alone. Spends excessively on food. Binges impulsively or eats continuously. Goes from one diet to the next. Eats little in public. Consumes large quantities of food in private. Participates in fewer social activities due to embarrassment over appearance.
ED-NOS (Eating Disorder—Not Otherwise Specified)	Doctors use this term for a variety of "unspecified" eating disorders: "ED-NOS" might refer to a woman, for example, who has anorexia, but who still menstruates, or whose weight is "normal." Or, perhaps, the term might identify some-one who purges without bingeing; who induces vomiting, for instance, after eating only a small quantity of food. In short, "ED-NOS" describes a combination of anorectic and bulimic features.	In these instances people are doing more than simply taking in too much or too little food—they are, clearly, in some kind of psychological pain, as well as being in danger of hurting themselves physically. Some people who have an ED-NOS practice chewing but not swallowing food; they simply spit it out. These "unspecified" eating disorders may not be as noticeable as others but can be just as hazardous.	Any kind of unhealthy eating pattern that is accompanied by disordered body perceptions or over-reactive emotions, whether it fits a standard definition of "eating disorder" or not.

- Bruised or callused knuckles and fingers caused by sticking the fingers in the mouth and down the throat to induce vomiting. Sore throat and/or swollen glands due to irritation from stomach acid during purging.

- Dry skin, brittle hair, and hair loss. Malnutrition and hormonal imbalances. Hair growth on the face, back, and arms (fine hair called lanugo). Hormonal imbalances.

Anorexia, Bulimia, Compulsive Overeating:
- Dental problems. Teeth and gum deterioration, decalcification of teeth and enamel loss, arthritis, osteoporosis, infertility, back pain, joint discomfort, poor circulation, heart problems, a feeling of weakness, sleep problems, exhaustion.

Binge Eating:
- A tendency to feel warm or hot, due to increased exertion placed on the body by excess weight and increased digestive activities.

- A fast and/or irregular heart rate. High blood pressure caused by increased weight gain and possible raised cholesterol levels.

- Joint pain caused by additional stresses on the body brought on by excess weight.

- Poor circulation due to constricted veins and arteries. Victims often tire easily.

- Exhaustion, decreased endurance, and dizziness brought on by increased stress on the body, nutritional imbalances, a fast heart rate, and high blood pressure.

- Varicose veins and spider veins, muscle soreness decreased mobility, hormonal imbalances.

Beyond normal

If so many types and degrees of eating disorders exist, what distinguishes a true disorder from eating habits that cross the line and exceed what our culture considers normal?

On the one hand, some professionals describe and diagnose eating disorders so exactly that people can brush aside their own dangerous habits. On the other hand, it may not be accurate to characterize someone who seems constantly absorbed by her own body shape and who exercises regularly as having an eating disorder.

Instead, detailed medical diagnoses should be considered in a broader context, taking into account not only specific disordered behaviors but also the wider pattern of a person's attitudes and habits and his psychological or environmental background.

As pointless and unhealthy as dieting may be for most of us, there is a difference between people who go on diets every once and a while and people who are perpetual dieters, especially those who demonstrate a strong need to control not only their own lives but also the lives of people around them. When constant efforts to control their diets fail, some people take out their frustration and disappointment on themselves. Or, they may blame others: "If you'd been there for me, I wouldn't have had to starve myself."

"Ordinary" dieters may get discouraged from time to time about their weight or appearance, but people who have eating disorders are pessimistic and negative about virtually every aspect of their lives. For example, people who have anorexia are rarely satisfied with any accomplishment, even if

Watch Out!
Even if you can't see direct evidence of an eating disorder, look for indirect clues, especially when you notice a preoccupation with food. Listen for statements such as, "I'm too fat," "I'm ugly," or "My life would be better if I just lost weight." Watch for evidence of low self-esteem and guilt in comments such as, "I never do anything right," or "nothing I ever do is enough." And take it seriously when a friend says he's fearful of being stared at or doesn't want to go somewhere because he just doesn't want to be seen.

they appear to be overachievers. While people who have anorexia may become withdrawn, people who have bulimia tend to be more outgoing. And although people who binge seem quite social in public, they generally suffer from feelings of embarrassment or humiliation in social settings. In particular, they fear being seen while eating in public; while purchasing groceries, diet pills or laxatives; or while purging—all are perceived as shameful behaviors by the person who has bulimia or a Binge Eating Disorder.

Reviewing all the symptoms and *possible* symptoms of eating disorders may create a confusing picture, but the professionals who treat these disorders use one rule of thumb in determining whether someone has an eating disorder:

If you suspect an eating disorder in yourself or someone close to you, there probably is one.

Just the Facts

- Eating disorders may be surprisingly hard to recognize.

- Personal denial and cultural attitudes toward dieting make it difficult to recognize some eating disorders.

- Not all disordered behavior patterns need to meet the full criteria of an eating disorder to qualify as a problem.

- Certain symptoms are unique to each disorder.

- If you suspect an eating disorder, it probably exists.

GET THE SCOOP ON...
How to approach an eating disorder
▪ What not to do ▪ What you can do
▪ When immediate action is necessary ▪ What
to do before treatment begins ▪ Getting help
for yourself and others

What to Do If Someone You Know Has an Eating Disorder

Chapter 9

If you suspect that someone you know has an eating disorder, or if you think you may have one yourself, you can explore the possibility in private and anonymously. Be sure to make contact with some of the resources listed at the back of this book (see Appendix B, "Resource Guide"). This is an important step toward recovery: To solve any problem, it's critical to acknowledge that there is one.

Gaining awareness

Many of the organizations listed in Appendix B offer information about where to get help for an eating disorder, but Web sites can be quite useful, too. Some of the personal stories posted in various sites go a long way toward dispelling some of the guilt and shame many people feel about their disorders.

Personal accounts on the Web do not offer treatment, of course, but they *can* provide a strong sense

Unofficially...
While it is understandable to feel like this, it is not productive: "She hurt me so much. I can't sleep at night worrying about how she is doing and how long she has to live. Why is she doing this to me?" The sufferer is not "doing" anything to hurt you on purpose—*she's* hurting. Taking action to ease the sufferer's path doesn't always make sense. Family members should seek treatment for themselves in order to learn how to manage the fears and anger that inevitably arise.

of camaraderie and underscore that the victim is not alone. This gives many people the courage to seek treatment in a more active way. Some Web sites also point the way to good sources of treatment.

Reading about other peoples' experiences with an eating disorder and asking questions anonymously may help you or someone you know realize that literally millions of others share the same kinds of fears and feelings. Gaining awareness that eating disorders are a health problem, not a source of shame or an indication of worth, can lead to positive actions and results.

Even if you *do* recognize that an eating disorder is not a statement about a person's character or moral fitness, you may be at a loss about what to do or how to help, and this frustration can lead to anger. It's all too easy to assume that the disordered behavior is willful rather than compulsive and that anger, punishment, or control will fix it.

At the same time, watching someone slowly starve, wear herself down with overexercise, or eat herself sick by gorging and purging can be excruciating. It's almost as painful to witness these eating disorders as it is to experience them in person.

How to relate to someone who has an eating disorder

According to some specialists, one of the best ways to relate to someone who has an eating disorder is to focus on something other than their weight. Practice acceptance—and no matter how you feel, try to avoid making negative comments. Instead, express your affection and emphasize the positive whenever you can:

- Keep your own food habits healthy, as an example to others. Being on a diet yourself will send a confusing message.

- Remember that the person who has an eating disorder needs to be in control of his own weight and eating habits.

- Be patient, gentle, but persistent about encouraging someone who has an eating disorder to seek professional help.

What doesn't work

No matter how much you may *want* someone who has anorexia or bulimia to get better, there are a few things you should avoid doing. For example, you cannot force someone who has anorexia to eat, stop someone who has bulimia from purging, or make someone who overeats compulsively stop overeating. In fact, the first thing to understand about eating disorders is that they are not about food. (See Chapter 3, "Our Relationship with Food," for details.)

If you are the parent of a child under the age of 18, you are responsible for his well-being, no matter how much he may fight or plead to be left alone. It is up to you to make sure that your child sees a doctor or goes to the hospital if it becomes apparent that he needs help. Never forget how serious an eating disorder is or how important it is to get early treatment. At all costs, avoid thinking of treatment as a simple matter of discipline. Rather, the issue is keeping your child safe from a debilitating physical and emotional condition.

Using force to push another adult into seeking help is just as useless and cruel as trying to bully a child. However, you *can* provide support and encouragement. Also learn as much as possible, not only about the disorder, but also about the friend, partner, or relative who has it.

Watch Out!
What if you have an eating disorder? If your family and friends are constantly telling you that you look too thin, if you feel embarrassed because you are eating far too much and secretly vomit or otherwise get rid of food, or if you prefer to eat in private because the amount of food you eat is so excessive, then you may be developing an eating disorder. Talk to your family, a trusted friend, or a doctor who will listen.

Choosing another approach

Instead of using negative force, a positive, gentle approach in which you discuss the facts and show your concern is more likely to work. People who have eating disorders are emotionally fragile and need to be handled with care. Instead of pushing at a person with cranky questions and negative observations such as "You look awful," or "Are you sick?," approach her with a caring statement, such as: "You've lost a lot of weight recently and I'm concerned about you." Or, say, "I'm here for you if you want to talk."

Anything you can say to communicate your affection and concern is more beneficial than a threatening "Would you just eat!" or "Stay out of the damn bathroom!" A person who has an eating disorder already has low self-esteem. Being critical or angrily apprehensive about her condition will only make it worse.

If you are close enough to a friend or relative who has an eating disorder, there's nothing wrong with inviting him to join you for dinner, a relaxed conversation, or any other pleasurable activity instead of laying on guilt with questions or statements such as "Why are you doing this to me?" or "Look at what you're doing to your family and friends!"

You may think that an angry, confrontational approach is the most direct way to help, but in fact it is a dangerously selfish one that puts an even greater burden on the person who is already suffering horribly from a compulsive disorder.

Likewise, don't plead or whine: "Why are you doing this to yourself?" Remember that people who have anorexia or bulimia do not choose to do this to themselves. Eating disorders are a coping

Unofficially...
No matter how "perfect" they may seem, research has shown that among individuals who have eating disorders, women in particular have poor coping skills. However, men who have eating disorders experience more difficulties than women in coping with stress.

mechanism, a means of dealing with depression, stress, and self-hate that have built up over many years. An eating disorder is a reflection of the pain some people feel inside. The best influence that a parent, partner, spouse, child, or friend can have on someone who is suffering in this way is to communicate a sense of hope. Optimism about the future and the results of good medical care can help galvanize someone who has a disorder into getting the treatment she so desperately needs.

Things you *can* do

Despite the frightening nature of some eating disorders, treatment is available and is successful. (For details about these treatments, see Chapter 10, "The Treatment Process.") It is up to each person who has an eating disorder to find the best treatment for herself, but you can help provide information and encouragement, too. Just let the person you care about know that there's something to fit her particular needs and that you will support her throughout her recovery.

Be direct

Often the best and most basic thing you can do for someone who has an eating disorder is to communicate your concerns directly, but in a nonjudgmental way. It will also make you feel better for having said what is on your mind without resorting to anger, guilt, or accusations.

Here's what professionals suggest:

1. Speak directly to the person who has an eating disorder. It's very common for people to consult with the friends and family of the person who has an eating disorder behind her back. This kind of evasion is both annoying and hurtful.

2. Stick to the facts. Tell the person that you're concerned about a particular behavior or pattern of behavior.

3. Don't get emotional or critical, but do express your concern honestly and clearly.

4. Encourage the person to seek treatment.

5. Help the person get to a physician, preferably one who knows something about eating disorders, for a physical exam, lab work, and an EKG. Even if the person who has a disorder denies the problem, he will probably respond to concerns about his physical health.

Be cautious

Be a good listener. Be gentle, caring, and not bossy to someone who has an eating disorder.

Don't tell the person what to do; just be encouraging.

Be patient once your friend has started to recover. The process can be very confusing and painful. It's not a straight road, and it can be a long one.

Don't overstep your boundaries. If the person has asked you not to do certain things or talk about them, don't.

Timesaver
Be clear about what you can control and what you can't. For instance, you can't force someone who has an eating disorder to "get better," but you *can* control how far you'll go to help.

Do not talk about food and weight, and don't keep asking the person about what he has or hasn't eaten, how much weight he has lost, or how good or bad he looks after gaining or losing weight. Don't be afraid to talk about your own experiences, but if you've never had a disorder yourself, don't pretend to understand. You can be wonderfully supportive without having lived through a similar experience yourself. It will be even more helpful to put the person in touch with others who are going through or who have already survived an eating disorder themselves.

Taking immediate action

Although people who suffer from eating disorders need to recover on their own, there are times when their state of health is imperiled and immediate medical attention or intervention is necessary. In these cases, you must take action. Find medical treatment immediately if a person exhibits any of the following signs:

- Dizziness, fatigue, fainting, blackouts
- Extreme temperature sensitivity
- Chest pains
- Tingling in the hands or feet
- Blood in the stools or vomit
- Stomach pains
- Incontinence
- Uncontrollable vomiting or diarrhea, and/or 10 percent or more weight loss

Remember that even if a person is desperate for help, he may be afraid to ask for it, especially if he doesn't feel deserving.

Stage by stage

Most people who have eating disorders go through several stages of awareness and acceptance of their condition. At each stage, they respond to different approaches to getting treatment.

Here's what's most likely to work at each stage:

Stage 1: Denial is at work in this stage. Here you're dealing with someone who completely refuses to acknowledge that she has a problem:

"My husband told me that he has an eating problem. He says he knows it makes him weak and tired, but he refuses to change anything. I can't say whether he likes being thin because he hides inside baggy clothes. Still, he sometimes says he loves being the way he is and is afraid of getting fat. I know his health has deteriorated in the last couple of weeks. He blames it on stress and is always tired. Sometimes he talks about feelings of depression. I don't think he has anorexia because he eats fatty foods sometimes and doesn't check his weight. But if he doesn't have anorexia, why does he refuse to eat regularly or gain weight? I told him I was worried about his health, but the only answer I ever get is 'I'm fine.' Can anybody help?"

As the partner, parent, or friend of someone who seems to have an eating disorder, it usually helps to get counseling on how to best address either denial or confusing symptoms.

- Express your concerns.
- Point out the facts.
- If she won't budge, suggest seeing a nutritionist who can recommend "safe foods" that might help round out her nutritional intake.
- Insist on a medical exam. Most people will respond to concerns about their physical health, even if they deny that there's an eating problem.

Stage 2: The person acknowledges there's a problem, but he doesn't want to change. ("I know I have eating problems, but I'm the thinnest I've ever been, and I feel great!")

- Suggest seeing a nutritionist (see the previous note).

- Suggest psychotherapy, not to change eating, but to address emotional issues underlying eating problems. Sometimes people are willing to start here.

- Insist on a medical exam.

Stage 3: The person acknowledges there's a problem and wants help.

This is an easy one.

Whatever the stage of denial or awareness, change *is* possible, even if it is slow. Still, it may help to know that the process has three stages: awareness, attitude, and action. According to the social scientists who came up with this formula, becoming aware that there *is* a problem ("Maybe I *am* eating oddly.") is essential to making any kind of progress. Next, they look for an attitude change ("I don't want to be sick all the time."). Finally, any successful action such as pursuing treatment comes from an open attitude.

Another pattern of change noted by social science researchers is abbreviated DREC, which stands for denial, resistance, exploration, and commitment. According to this analysis, the person who has an eating disorder may blankly deny any problem: "Why should I get treatment when I don't have a problem?" Then, rabid resistance to the idea of change might even be seen as a sign of progress: "No way will I cut back on exercise!" Exploration could occur when the person who has the eating disorder actually reads the brochures you offer or clicks on to an anorexia chat room. Commitment might come later, it is hoped, when treatment has begun.

Unofficially...
Patients who have bulimia often improve over time. The results of a recent Harvard study indicate that over the long term, individuals who have bulimia often do improve. Of the 173 women in the study, 46.8 percent were in full remission from bulimia 10 years after diagnosis, and 23.1 percent had achieved partial remission. However, 30 percent of the women diagnosed with bulimia more than 10 years earlier continued to suffer from binge eating or purging.

Reading matters

The fact that you are reading this book shows that you are interested in more information. You can find a lot more fact-based material from the Web sites and groups listed in Appendix B, as well as in other sections of this book. As the parent, spouse, partner, or friend of someone who has an eating disorder, you can gather material—including a list of nearby treatment centers—and give it to him. But always approach this person with this attitude: "You know I'm worried. It would make me feel better if you would a take a look at this material."

As the parent, partner, or friend of someone who has an eating disorder, it is completely appropriate for you to discuss the matter with your family doctor, school counselor, or workplace employee assistance program. These professionals might be able to reach the person you love, if that's what seems appropriate. Or, from these expert sources you might receive guidance about how best to handle the situation, what danger signals to watch for, and how to handle your own feelings about the situation. In some cases, it is advisable to make an intervention: to gather several people who matter in the sufferer's life and, with professional backing, confront her in a concerned, nonthreatening fashion while offering a plan for treatment.

Blunting a disorder's dangerous effects

What if you can't persuade the person you care about to get the treatment he needs, no matter what you do? Or, what if you are not ready to take the next step toward recovery, if you have an eating disorder yourself? Eating-disorder specialists point out that there *are* steps to take, short of treatment, to mediate the effects of an eating disorder. While you or someone you know is getting ready to begin treatment, doctors suggest the following tips:

- Drink lots of fluids to ward off dehydration.

- Take vitamin and mineral supplements for nutritional support without adding calories.

- The use of diuretics (and other forms of purging) can create serious electrolyte imbalances; if you must use diuretics, be sure to eat potassium-rich foods (such as bananas). Add fitness bars or shakes to your diet, if you can, to provide at least some nutrition.

- Rinse your mouth with an antacid after vomiting to reduce damage to the throat, esophagus, and tooth enamel.

- Switch from stimulant laxatives to bulk laxatives, such as Metamusil or Fiber Con, and drink lots of water while taking them. These won't upset the fluid balance of the body the way stimulant laxatives do and are a safe way to come off laxatives.

- To cut down on bingeing, try eating small amounts of food every three hours.

- To try to accept your body, focus on one good thing you can find about it, and stop reading fashion and fitness magazines.

- Get a thorough physical exam, including a full set of blood tests and an EKG heart-function test. Stay in close touch with your doctor to take care of any physical problems the disorder may trigger.

These suggestions are not treatments, of course. Rather, they are simple stopgaps—methods of

Watch Out!
Emetics, such as ipecac are extremely dangerous and may cause nerve or muscle damage with frequent use. Avoid them.

Watch Out!
Diet pills are toxic in large doses. If you must, use them only according to instructions. In case of a medical emergency, people close to you should alert medical personnel to the possibility a of diet-pill overdose.

dealing with a few aspects of an eating disorder before real help comes in the form of professional treatment.

Getting into treatment

Getting treatment for someone who restricts food or who binges or purges can be very difficult. After all, if this person could cope with psychological and emotional distress, he wouldn't need to use food as a means of distraction.

Sometimes when the sufferer is secretly ready to let go of her disorder, it just takes the urging of a friend to motivate the first step toward treatment. For example, a roommate might offer an informational pamphlet and express the wish that it be read. Or, a spouse might make an appointment with the family physician on the pretext that it is just an annual checkup. But it is not always so easy to get some friends or relatives into treatment.

Convincing someone to get help may take the careful intervention of other family members, friends, and professionals. Very often the sufferer is willing to go to a non–eating disorder specialist—a skin doctor or dentist, perhaps—to be treated for some of the side effects that have resulted from an eating disorder. Or, someone who is already in recovery might persuade your friend or loved one to go to a support group meeting "just to try it out." If someone in your family is in therapy, his therapist might request that the whole family come in for a session and take it from there. Or, it may take emergency hospitalization for a medical crisis that resulted from the disorder to get someone within reach of treatment. In the meantime, the loved ones of the victim are suffering.

> **"**
> I have been aware that I suffer from bulimia for the past eight years. I have decided to finally seek help because this obsession has been such a big part of my life, but I've found that I can't stop. In fact, I have added diet pills and alcohol to the things I take.
> —A young man who started purging as a college athlete
> **"**

Getting help

All the suggestions made so far can be helpful to the person who has anorexia, bulimia, or Binge Eating Disorder. But what about *you*? What if you live with someone who suffers from one of these disorders? The experience may be causing you and the rest of your family more pain than you realize.

Helping yourself

No matter how strong your desire may be to help a suffering friend or a member of the family, the need for you, the helper, to get support is at least as strong. For one thing, you can be a lot more helpful if you have a solid understanding of the disorder.

At the same time, it's important for you to realize that no matter how much you know, there is only so much you can do to help someone who has an eating disorder. You can point the way, but you can't force a cure. The pain and frustration of trying to live someone else's life destroys the helper's life as well. So, it's vital for many reasons to find help for yourself.

As a friend or relative of someone who has an eating disorder, support is available to you on the same Web sites and electronic bulletin boards that are suggested for people who have eating disorders (see the list of resources in Appendix B).

Here are a few examples of the kind of support and advice you can find, offer, or ask for on the Internet:

> "I just need someone to listen! I have written some e-mails to people on this site, and I find it's good to get support and send it to others in the same situation. I am continually looking for answers and try to do more research whenever I get the time. If anyone has found

"
She's in therapy and on antidepressants for her depression. Meanwhile, I think I am going to go crazy trying to figure out what to do.
—The mother of a woman in her 20s who suffers from anorexia
"

Moneysaver
Most of the Web sites that are related to eating disorders in Appendix B have chat rooms for family and friends of people who have eating disorders.

Timesaver
One thing that family and friends can learn from the treatment they get themselves is how futile and even self-defeating it is to do too much for someone who has an eating disorder. This kind of enabling is more than a waste of time; it can make the situation a great deal worse.

any answers or something that has helped them or their loved one, I'd be more than happy to hear it. I send lots of love to everyone."

"Now that she is getting help, it is difficult to let go of the desire to help. I try not to, but it is hard, and there is no one who really understands what I mean. Having found this excellent Web site, I hope that someone out there who can relate to this or offer words of advice will contact me. Thank you for listening...."

"I know the pain that we siblings go through waiting for recovery. I'm willing to listen to or share stories with anyone who contacts me."

"No matter what your family situation is or how many times you've been set aside, always remember: You're important, too. Stay strong."

At the very least, you can get lots of practice sharing your concerns and experiences on the Internet. You'll also find "live" groups and treatment sources where you can get almost as much support for yourself as the person who actually has an eating disorder.

All the careful handling in the world may or may not help get a person who has an eating disorder into treatment. (Details on treatment begin in the next chapter.) In any case, it's clear that the people who are closest to the victims of eating disorders suffer greatly and need a lot of care themselves.

Being there: Living with someone who has an eating disorder

No one can describe the pain of being close to someone who has a serious eating disorder more eloquently than the people who love her:

"My older sister has a severe case of bulimia.
I don't want her to die, but at the same time,
I am frustrated because my life has been so
painfully disrupted by her disorder. I feel like
I'm her older sister or even her mother. I feel
guilty about being angry that she is sick, but
at the same time it is so emotionally, spiritu-
ally, and mentally draining to live with her
and to love her...."

"My 22-year-old sister has bulimia. She's older
than me by two years, and we are both at university, away from home. My parents asked
me to move in with her this year to keep an
eye on her, but to be honest, after almost five
months of it I can't handle it any more. I try
to be understanding and I know she has
problems, but in some ways I just feel so
angry at her. I'm only 20, and I'm trying to
find my own way in the world, and I can't
take this responsibility...."

"We have taken our daughter to over a dozen
different rehabs. She's been in the emergency room over two dozen times and has
been resuscitated three times. Sometimes she
seems to respond to treatment, then slips
back. Her weight got down to less than 60
pounds when she was 15. She's almost 20
now, and it seems to be getting better. She's
gaining weight now and eating. We try not to
get our hopes up, though...."

A single eating disorder can send spasms of pain
through an entire network of concerned people. The
friends and families of people who have eating disorders may not have *physical* symptoms themselves,
but their suffering can be profound. Treatment for

eating disorders can help you and others, not just the primary victims of eating disorders.

Just the Facts

- People who are close to those who suffer from eating disorders need to communicate their concerns carefully but directly.

- Resources are available to help you communicate effectively with someone who has an eating disorder.

- Web sites offer easy access to support.

- Subtle signs from a person who has an eating disorder can show you the best way to help her get into treatment.

- You can do lots of things to ameliorate your condition—or someone else's—before you begin treatment for an eating disorder.

- People who are close to victims of eating disorders can find much needed help for themselves, too.

Treatments for
Eating Disorders

GET THE SCOOP ON...
What the treatments are ▪ The therapeutic
process ▪ Tailoring therapy to the individual ▪
Stumbling blocks ▪ What recovery feels like

PART IV

The Treatment Process

Eating disorders may be pervasive, stubborn, and dangerous, but they *are* highly treatable. This reality, however, is very often lost in highly emotionalized media portrayals of eating disorders. In fact, the greatest stumbling blocks to treatment are exactly the sort of misconceptions that are so often exploited and fostered by the media. Likewise, fear that treatment is harsh can impede progress, when the fact is that successful therapy is gentle and gradual. It is especially important for people who have anorexia to know this because their intense fear of gaining weight can keep them from getting treatment.

The treatment of eating disorders has undergone many changes over the past several decades, and therapeutic approaches continue to adapt both to new information about the nature of eating disorders and to developments in the surrounding culture. In the early 1980s, for example, a much more medical approach often involving lengthy hospitalization was adopted once an eating disorder was

131

taken seriously enough to warrant professional attention.

More recently, however, the high costs and difficulties of that treatment, combined with the results of research and professional experience with eating disorders, have led to different therapeutic techniques. Despite the fact that certain patterns are similar from one eating disorder to another, the prevailing approach now is to consider each patient as unique. Therefore, treatment is tailored to meet individual needs. To accomplish this, a specialist or a group of specialists works with each patient.

This chapter provides general information about treatments and how they work. The chapters that follow offer suggestions on how to find the most appropriate therapy, evaluate alternatives, and maintain health over the long term.

An overview of treatments

Unofficially... Teams aren't always necessary for successful treatment. In fact, many people are treated by individual therapists who specialize in eating disorders.

Because eating disorders stem from complex physical, psychological, medical, and social roots, their treatment often calls for a combination of approaches that involves physicians, psychotherapists, pharmacologists, and nutritionists working individually or as a team. Even if therapy is initiated during a hospital stay, the patient also can benefit from the support of family and friends.

Each treatment plan is individualized. For example, someone who has occasional purging problems but no physical symptoms might need an initial checkup with a physician and then might see only a therapist. Or, someone who strictly limits food intake might need to see a therapist only. Other people, however, need to be encouraged to eat and to give up food rules. In these cases, regular consultations with a psychotherapist would in all likelihood speed recovery.

Some people are more comfortable working with their own physician once they have been able to admit a problem and accept help. This treatment can be successful if the doctor is well versed in dealing with eating disorders. A physician with less expertise would be wise to consult a specialist even if the patient does not wish to seek other therapy.

Depending on the specifics of a patient's condition, treatment can be successful after a fairly brief series of sessions with a therapist, or it can take longer or require more intense multidisciplinary attention. Most patients find long-term follow-up valuable, perhaps in the form of professional therapy or support groups, or simply by employing techniques learned during treatment.

Methods of treatment

Methods of treatment include some or all of the following:

- Medical treatment in a hospital, as an outpatient or in a controlled residential setting

- Individual psychotherapy or psychiatric treatment, incorporating a variety of schools and approaches

- Group therapy

- Couples or family therapy

- Nutritional counseling

- Pharmacotherapy

To be effective, each therapeutic approach must provide both the patient and his family with what professionals call education. This means explaining to the patient what is happening and why at every stage of treatment. Education is a critical part of fully involving the patient in his recovery, and it

66

You have to find the way that's best for you. But you can't recover unless you want to and are willing to do whatever it takes to get better. For me, recovery meant weeks in the hospital, following a rigid food plan designed by a nutritionist, going to outpatient therapy, getting involved with support groups, and reading books. Plus, feeling positive. I started small and focussed on just one thing I liked about my body. I built on, that and eventually I found happiness and recovery.
—A young woman who has worked her way through the process of recovery

99

Moneysaver
Treatment need not go on indefinitely once symptoms have abated and you are feeling better. In fact, it is possible to continue treatment on your own outside of therapy after you've learned how to use a few helpful techniques.

builds a foundation of information that will make it possible for a patient to make significant changes in food- and weight-related behavior. Topics that are covered initially include: the physiology of starvation, the dangers of purging, how dieting backfires, the psychological compulsions behind destructive food-related behavior, and a presentation of how and why body perceptions become distorted.

Patients are often surprised at the harm they are doing to their bodies or by the fact that their patterns of thought and behavior are common to many other people. Education also helps patients examine their own food-related habits and beliefs. The educational phase of treatment is critical because it breaks down denial, dispels the patient's sense of isolation, and encourages her active participation in the process of recovery.

Nutritional therapists, 12-step support groups, behavioral psychologists, and insight-oriented psychiatrists all find it valuable to educate patients about the basics of nutrition and the results of disordered eating patterns.

How the treatments work

The ultimate goal of each kind of therapy is to restore order to eating patterns, though each may vary in approach. The following is an overview of the various types of therapy employed in the treatment of eating disorders. Please note that this overview does not represent a *progression* of treatment, but it presents a variety of approaches, one or more of which might be used. (Details about individual therapies are provided later in this chapter.) The level of therapeutic intensity depends upon the specific nature of the disorder and the condition of the patient.

First level of intensity in treatment: The first level involves outpatient psychotherapy. This involves visiting a therapist's office once or twice a week and might include group, couples, or family therapy. Most people can be successfully treated at this least-intensive level of treatment.

Second level of intensity in treatment: This level involves daily therapy for people whose symptoms continue despite outpatient treatment. Day treatment programs involve day-long or sometimes all-evening sessions that include one or two meals, group therapy, and possibly family therapy before the patient goes home at night. This level of treatment helps give patients greater control over their symptoms than the first. In fact, many people are able to successfully change eating patterns in day treatment programs. These programs are also cheaper and less intrusive than in-patient hospitalization programs offered by hospitals.

Third level of intensity in treatment: In-patient hospitalization is necessary at this stage for people who need more than day treatment. This involves being admitted to a hospital where medical personnel can manage and monitor eating problems. Some programs for eating disorders are housed in psychiatric hospitals and require patients to be medically stable before they are admitted simply because the facilities are not equipped to handle complicated medical emergencies. Therefore, a patient may need to be admitted to a hospital first before entering some

Timesaver
Once someone is willing to deal with an eating disorder—and learn everything there is to know about it—the treatment of it is that much more effective. Points to understand include: bodily responses to starvation, abnormal and normal hunger, a healthy weight range, minimum food intake needed to stabilize weight and metabolic rate, optimal food intake for health, the concept of a set point for weight, and the way in which food- and weight-related behaviors change during the process of recovery.

programs for eating disorders. In-hospital visits for treatment can last anywhere from a week to several months. Because treatment is around-the-clock, it allows maximum control of symptomatic behaviors.

Long-term treatment: Sometimes following an in-patient stay a person chooses to have residential treatment, which involves long-term care in a residential setting. This form of non-medical rehabilitation allows people to continue with monitored eating, group and individual psychotherapy, and educational activities that help them manage their disorders. Residential treatment usually offers more flexibility than a hospital and is geared more toward assisting the person to live independently. These programs, which are well known for the treatment of substance abuse, can also be tremendously helpful as halfway houses that provide a safe transition from hospitals to independent life.

Other areas of specialty are often brought into the treatment process:

Nutritional counseling: This involves seeing a nutritionist, sometimes weekly or sometimes less frequently, for a one-time consultation. The nutritionist assesses the person's weekly food intake and suggests nutritious foods to balance her diet and perhaps to work toward a more acceptable weight range. In an effort to dispel distorted thoughts about food, nutritional counselors educate people about how food actually affects the body. For example, some people don't understand that the body needs food from every food group to stay

Unofficially...
The psychonutritional approach to the treatment of eating disorders is one in which psychotherapy and medical nutrition therapy are combined to assist recovery.

healthy, or they believe that fat produces fat and therefore eat only "safe" foods, such as plain protein or greens.

Psychopharmacology: Sometimes medication is an important adjunct to psychotherapy, especially if the patient has another illness, such as depression or Obsessive Compulsive Disorder (OCD). Very often medication can help manage symptoms more effectively. The first step is assessment by a psychiatrist, who may prescribe an antidepressant or an antianxiety medication. If the psychiatrist happens to be the person's therapist, he will be able to prescribe medication during regular sessions. If the therapist is not a psychiatrist, he will refer the person to one. If a psychiatrist is prescribing medication only, he will see the person once a week for the first month or so and then as infrequently as once every three months for checkups. If several trials of different medications are required, more frequent psychiatry visits will be needed.

Medical Management: This means seeing an internist (a medical doctor) for physical checkups, lab work, weight checks, and so on. Ideally, the internist should be familiar with eating disorders. In any case, the doctor's role is to determine what physical problems have developed as a result of a disorder and to monitor the patient medically with physical exams, lab tests, and perhaps weight checks. How often a person needs to see an internist depends on the severity of the problem. Once a patient is medically stabilized,

Watch Out!
If a child or adolescent who has an eating disorder needs medication, a child psychiatrist will not only know about psychiatric medications, but more importantly, he or she will know about the differential physical and psychological effects of therapeutic drugs on children and teenagers.

physicians are not usually a necessary part of treatment, unless other therapists see the need for additional or ongoing medical input.

Some people who have eating disorders receive the attention of an entire team of professionals at some point in their treatment. Even where a total-team approach may not be needed, individual therapists can and do work together. For example, if a person with an eating disorder is also depressed or knows that she requires medication, she may want a psychiatrist to be her therapist so that the psychiatrist will be able to prescribe medication during her regular sessions. However, psychiatrists are the most expensive of mental health professionals. If the expense prohibits that choice, it is very common to see a psychologist or social worker and to visit a psychiatrist only occasionally. Therapists usually refer their patients to psychiatrists with whom they work closely, which generally means that treatment is greatly enhanced by both of their efforts.

Treatment goals

The specifics of each approach to treating eating disorders may differ, but the primary goal for treating all types of eating disorders can be summed up simply: to normalize eating patterns and establish and maintain a healthy body weight.

Emergency treatment

Although hospitalization is not common for most eating disorders, treatment may begin in a hospital—especially for anorexia—because sometimes the first goal of treatment is to stabilize or even save a life.

Hospitalization is more common for people who have anorexia, especially those who purge, than it is

---

The Goals of Therapy for Eating Disorders:

1. Restoration of a healthy body weight

2. Development of normal eating behavior

3. Development of social comfort and nutritional balance in eating situations

4. Treatment of psychiatric disorders related to eating problems

5. Establishment of an appropriate exercise program

6. Restoration of accurate body perceptions and a positive sense of identity

7. Treatment of medical complications connected with disorders

8. Improved family and interpersonal relationships

9. Aftercare plans for treatment and prevention of relapse

---

for people who have bulimia because these people put themselves in greater physical danger. Professionals make decisions to hospitalize a patient for treatment based on his physical and mental condition. One of the most important factors they consider is the amount of weight lost. If the person is about 15–20 percent below healthy weight, she usually requires hospitalization, especially if weight loss has occurred swiftly and persistently, despite therapy.

Hospitalization is necessary in most cases where there are serious physical problems, such as diabetes and certain heart irregularities, or when a mental dysfunction, such as depression, puts a

Watch Out!
When someone who has an eating disorder is in treatment and still suffers from symptoms and continued weight loss—or when that person refuses or doesn't succeed in out-patient treatment—hospitalization *must* be considered.

patient in danger. Lack of response to outpatient treatment programs or absence of a helpful home environment may result in hospitalization as well.

In the hospital

Although lab tests taken by people who have been hospitalized for eating disorders may point to serious conditions, they are usually the results of dehydration and starvation. Patients begin to return to normal as soon as fluids and nutrition are introduced intravenously or through tube feeding. As soon as possible, however, patients must be encouraged to eat regular, if small, meals. Mealtimes are supervised by medical staff, who also make an effort to ensure that patients do not purge.

While in-depth psychological therapy is not likely to be practiced in the hospital, reward systems are used to encourage eating, and the patient's involvement in her own treatment begins early. Although weight gain is the primary goal for people who have anorexia, it's important for the patients to understand that gaining weight is just the *beginning* of therapy and that they must actively plan and participate in choices about their own recovery.

Weight gain can be very frightening for people who have eating disorders (especially those who have anorexia), so a workable plan for gaining weight needs to be developed gently, with the patient's cooperation rather than through the use of force. For example, a doctor may set a goal of achieving as little as 90 percent to as much as 115 percent of the patient's ideal weight before he or she can be discharged from the hospital. However, it is vital for the patient to cooperate in achieving the goal, both as a practical matter and as a learning experience. Successful hospital programs teach patients not just about the nature of their disorder, but also what they are actually *doing* to themselves and how they can affect the future in a positive way.

Residential treatment

During a hospital stay, physiological and psychiatric evaluations can help determine whether a patient's biochemical or emotional condition requires specialized treatment. Some patients may need closer follow-up than others do. For example, a patient may eat just enough to get out of the hospital, and even begin to feel better emotionally as a result. Without ongoing support, however, she is especially vulnerable to relapse. For a patient like this, a longer stay in the structured environment of a residential treatment center is invaluable, especially if her family life is not supportive or is even destructive.

In the past, some residential treatments included shocking and frightening methods, such as allowing patients to eat until they became nauseated; patients were then asked to concentrate on their discomfort and write down their thoughts and feelings. During this agonizing process, bathrooms were kept locked so that patients would feel too ashamed to vomit without a private place to do so.

The effectiveness of these extreme methods has been vigorously disputed and repudiated by most professionals. In any case, patients should not fear them now. Therapy for eating disorders has come a long way since the era of forced public vomiting. Having said that, however, it is important nonetheless to ask about the techniques that are used at any residential center or program before entering it.

Tailoring therapy to the individual

Recent approaches to the treatment of eating disorders recognize that the very prospect of changing

Unofficially...
If practical or financial considerations make only a short hospital stay possible, a moderate weight gain (90 percent of the patient's normal weight) may have to be accepted as the next best goal for a patient who has anorexia. Under these circumstances, close follow-up care in an outpatient clinic is absolutely required.

eating patterns is in itself so frightening for most people with disorders that scary police tactics are not only redundant—they can even backfire. This kind of fear keeps some people away from getting help, which is a pity; the fact is that the willing cooperation and involvement of the patient is a huge component of successful treatment. Someone who doesn't want treatment, of course, won't make use of it.

Regardless, it is the responsibility of those who are in charge of the patient's care to go out of their way to involve the patient and to make sure that she receives a full range of treatment. For example, a therapist who takes a behavioral approach to treatment nevertheless may require medical specialists to establish a patient's physical condition. This therapist also might rely on a dietitian to provide nutritional guidance and support. Or, the therapist might consult a psychiatrist if she believes that depression might be part of a problem that could be alleviated with medication.

Once these experts set psychological and physical goals, the patient needs to see firsthand how psychological, medical, dietary, and social factors all play a part in recovery.

Unofficially...
A critical member of the treatment team is the patient. A patient's attitude and willingness to recover can make all the difference in a successful treatment.

Entering treatment

To a certain extent, the details of treatment depend on how it begins. Naturally, a patient seeking help for an eating disorder can choose which type of therapy seems most comfortable. However, some people take a much less direct route to getting treatment: In many of these cases, they don't seek help *specifically* for their disorder. Instead, they visit a professional for some other problem that ostensibly has nothing to do with eating disorders.

On the other hand, a person may visit a specialist in eating disorders on his own, knowing that he has a problem and that he is willing to face it. Other people are brought to a doctor or an eating specialist by a parent or someone close to them. Either way, an individual's own level of willingness to get better strongly affects the prognosis and becomes one of the challenges of any kind of treatment. If the patient hasn't come voluntarily, he may take longer to get with the program offered by a therapist. (This does not mean that parents or spouses should not bring loved ones into treatment; sometimes that very act of caring is a turning point for the patient.) Treatment can't be forced on anyone, of course, but a skilled therapist can find ways to elicit a patient's cooperation once she is in treatment.

One reason why it is so vital for professionals, as well as the general public, to know about eating disorders is that quite often an eating disorder is the underlying condition of a seemingly unrelated problem.

For example, an individual might visit a physician for any number of distressing physical symptoms such as hair loss, digestive difficulties, or skin troubles. All of these might seem unrelated, unless one has been sensitized and educated to see the connection between these kinds of symptoms and eating disorders. An experienced dentist who recognizes the deleterious effects of bulimia on teeth enamel, for example, will be alerted to the possibility of an eating disorder if one of his patients is seriously afflicted with cavities and other dental problems.

Whether it is a nutritionist who is sought for help with a diet, a psychotherapist for assistance

Timesaver
A professional who suspects an eating disorder in a patient who is seeking some other kind of help needs to explore the possibility by asking specific questions about forbidden foods, food rules, episodes of restriction, bingeing, purging, and the like.

with depression, or a school counselor for a solution to fatigue that interferes with schoolwork, each of these professionals should be alert to the possibility of an eating disorder. They must also be prepared to guide those who come to them for assistance into appropriate treatment.

Step by step

Regardless of approach, the first step toward successful treatment is accurate assessment. For example, Angela, an 18-year-old college student, went to a counseling center on campus at the urging of her roommate. There counselors took her history and determined that her physical condition was serious enough to warrant hospitalization. Another student, Cynthia, made an appointment with a nutritionist specifically to find a diet that works. Judging that a new diet was not what Cynthia needed, the nutritionist referred her to a physician for treatment of an eating disorder.

Assessment involves careful diagnosis of the specifics of a disorder (if there is one), as well as necessary physiological tests or perhaps a psychiatric evaluation. When someone visits a health professional with a problem that arouses suspicion of an eating disorder, initial interviews should include comments or a question or two about possible eating concerns, such as: "Do you have any concerns about food or eating?" or, "Our society today is so diet-conscious—do you ever go on diets or worry about weight?" Or, the interviewer may ask for a sample of a typical day's food intake, from the time the person gets up to when she goes to bed. If any foods are excluded, the interviewer may ask why—reasons such as food allergies, lactose intolerance, or vegetarianism often mask an eating disorder.

Given the serious possibility of a disorder, questions might also probe weight history and symptoms such as purging or irregular menstrual periods.

If an eating disorder is diagnosed, a treatment plan is then devised to address physiological and psychological issues in whatever priority is indicated. Professionals can determine which of the two aspects of treating eating disorders—restoring normal eating behaviors and addressing the underlying emotional issues—needs the most focus, at least initially.

Psychotherapy

A frequently employed psychological approach to treating eating disorders is Cognitive Behavioral Therapy (CBT). Developed by Dr. Christopher Fairburn at Oxford University in England, CBT is the most researched method of treating bulimia and binge eating problems and is currently one of the most successful. Adaptations of this method of treatment, which seeks to change disordered behavior, are being developed for people who have anorexia as well.

For patients who want to change their eating patterns, CBT may prove sufficient by itself. But in many cases, especially during the later stages of recovery, more traditional types of psychotherapy, such as "insight therapy," are used. Psychoanalysis and other types of "talking therapy" are instrumental in unearthing underlying psychological and emotional conflicts once CBT has relieved the active symptoms of an eating disorder. Because the initial aim of CBT is to improve eating patterns, therapists often work with dietitians and other medical professionals as well.

Cognitive Behavioral Therapy Divided into Three Stages

In the first stage, the main emphasis is on educating the patient about the mechanisms that maintain an eating disorder. Behavioral techniques are used to replace binge eating with a pattern of regular eating.

In stage 2, further emphasis on eating regularly—without dieting—is combined with cognitive procedures that bring the thoughts, beliefs, and values that maintain a disorder into sharper focus.

Stage 3 considers relapse prevention strategies.

Cognitive Behavior Therapy (CBT)

The theory behind the effectiveness of CBT is that triggers to bingeing are both physical and emotional. If a patient is hungry and has an emotional upset, there is little chance of her resisting the urge to binge. However, if the patient is satisfied—satiated, or feeling full—she may be able to use a coping strategy other than eating to manage stress. Therefore, in CBT, physical triggers are eliminated first through establishing a pattern of regular eating. Once overeating has become an intermittent rather than regular activity for the patient, emotional and thinking triggers are addressed by helping the patient to identify, question, and modify thoughts, beliefs, and attitudes that are relevant to the disorder. Finally, plans to maintain progress are discussed.

In CBT, patients keep records of their food intake and use workbooks and other tools to set goals for each week of treatment. Therapists use techniques that question and challenge patients' distorted food beliefs and provide practical help in developing new coping strategies to manage difficult emotions. A CBT therapist may ask a patient to articulate the half-conscious, automatic thoughts that might be ruling her life; then she may encourage the patient to question them himself. For example, the patient may say that he feels fat, but when asked to describe people of his own size and shape, he describes them as "too thin." The therapist then helps the patient to recognize the inconsistencies in his perceptions of himself and others.

Other psychological approaches to eating disorders

To involve patients in their own recovery, therapists explain the treatment they intend to use and tell how therapy will proceed. If the treatment is to be successful, it is essential for both patient and therapist to agree on it.

Therapists find that it is also beneficial to explain other approaches and to give patients the opportunity to choose from them. Not only is this an ethical and professional approach, but it also enlists the patient in her own recovery. For example, although a CBT professional takes a very different approach from that of a 12-step program (such as the one used by Overeaters Anonymous), the therapist needs to present the approach to his patient as an option or as an adjunct to treatment. (The 12-step programs differ from CBT in that they are based on abstinence—not eating foods that are troublesome or that may trigger a binge. CBT proposes that all kinds of food may be eaten, but only in moderation.)

"
To get over overeating, you need to start listening to your body. As simple as it sounds, it's the only way to change your habits once and for all. If you're hungry, eat. When you're full, stop. Remembering these two simple rules puts you on the road to healthy eating for the rest of your life.
—A young woman in recovery from an eating disorder, sharing her "secret"

> **❝**
> One of the things we must learn to do is find better ways to cope with our emotions. We have learned that eating too much or too little is a good way to block emotions. It is much easier to think about eating, not eating, eating too much, or how many calories we just had or will avoid... than it is to deal with our feelings and emotions.
> —A patient in recovery from an eating disorder
> **❞**

Another approach to treating eating disorders involves interpersonal or insight-oriented psychotherapy. This method doesn't address eating behaviors at all, but it focuses on underlying issues instead. Restricting, bingeing, and purging behaviors are seen as symbols of emotional deprivation and unmet needs. Relationships are carefully analyzed, therefore, to help the person discover ways in which her emotional needs are not being met and how this can be corrected.

There is also a feminist model of psychotherapy, an approach that helps women explore and recognize ways in which gender (being female) has predisposed them to eating disorders. According to the feminist model, eating disorders symbolize the degree to which conflicting role demands have affected the female experience. The approach supports women's needs to integrate the disparate parts of themselves into more powerful, whole persons who can make themselves heard.

Some therapists mix approaches. For example, CBT, which can be used to help bring patients' eating behaviors under control, might be combined with various techniques borrowed from psychoanalysis and other insight therapies to explore relationships and social stressors.

Some, but not all, patients benefit from group or family therapy. Where there is mutual trust—and where support is positive—these forms of therapy are valuable, but in some circumstances they can be detrimental. (See Chapter 11, "Selecting Treatment," for more details.)

Drug therapies

As we learn more about the biochemical causes of a variety of disorders, the temptation is to assume that there must be a pill to cure eating disorders. While there's no magic pill, some drug therapy is available, but experts use it with great care.

For example, the use of medicines to stimulate appetite in patients who have anorexia is generally not helpful because, in the end, it is the patients' emotions that are disordered, not their appetite. And, of course, the main idea behind treating anorexia is to encourage patients to normalize eating patterns. Drugs that cause weight gain aren't especially useful either because patients who have anorexia are usually reluctant to take them. What's more, the side effects can be uncomfortable or even dangerous to their enfeebled bodies. Indeed, no medications exist for treating anorexia, per se, although an antidepressant or antianxiety medicine may be prescribed if a patient is depressed or excessively anxious about certain food-related issues.

However, some medications may have a beneficial effect on Binge Eating Disorder and bulimia, especially those that relieve depression by boosting serotonin levels. (Research has shown that there is an imbalance of this brain chemical in people who have bulimia. This medication has not been proven to be thoroughly effective, and the results vary from person to person, so care needs to be taken when considering it and all other biochemical approaches to eating disorders.

Feeling full

No matter how sophisticated pharmaceutical treatments may become, successful therapy for eating disorders focuses on much more basic matters, such as helping patients learn when they are hungry and when they are full. Odd as this may sound to someone who has never experienced this, patients who have established restrictive eating patterns often stop experiencing the sensation of hunger. Because of this, hunger can no longer function as a cue for them to eat. These individuals must use a clock, not subjective feelings of hunger, to dictate mealtimes. The sensation of hunger returns after a more normal pattern of eating has been established.

Patients who restrict their intake of food often complain of bloating or excessive fullness after eating. Physiologically, this may be due to delayed gastric emptying. In other words, food from the previous day is sometimes found in the stomachs of patients who restrict food or binge. Psychologically, the feeling of fullness may result from anxiety about food intake or weight gain. Patients may become hypervigilant about certain body sensations, such as the feel of a snug waistband or gas pains.

Patients who binge may have difficulty feeling sated or full. Carbohydrates and fats have been found to trigger feelings of satiety, the sense that one has eaten enough. Patients who restrict fats, in particular, may not be able to "turn off" their stomachs, which can result in bingeing episodes a short time after eating. Although some patients who have bulimia may experience rebound hunger after eating high-fat, high-carbohydrate meals, most do not. Therefore, it is better to encourage consumption of sufficient amounts of fats and carbohydrates to trigger satiety, thus eliminating the physical triggers to bingeing.

Dealing with the scale

Patients who have eating disorders are strongly urged not to weigh themselves unless they wish to do so on a limited basis—say, once a week and under the supervision of a therapist. Weighing themselves

---

Key Points in Understanding Recovery

Patients who have eating disorders usually need to alter their attitudes and feelings about weight. Here are some points that are stressed in therapy:

1. Women's weight normally goes up and down within a range of about 6 pounds, regardless of food intake.

2. A patient should postpone choosing a specific weight range until she has regained control over eating.

3. Getting to a chosen weight range should not necessitate anything more than a few dietary restraints.

4. In most cases, returning to regular eating doesn't result in large increases in weight. Some people lose weight because it decreases binges or speeds up their metabolism, while other people's weight remains the same.

5. Most desired weights are arbitrary. A number doesn't mean anything in itself, yet people attach great significance to numbers. For instance, some people feel that round numbers such as 110, 120, and 130 are better than non-round numbers such as 118, 122, and 139.

---

under these circumstances can be instructive and important to some patients, if only because it demonstrates that their ideas are mistaken about how certain foods are "dangerous" to their weight.

Unofficially...
During CBT, improvement goals are based on a patient's food charts and habits, and they may include directions such as: "Eat every three hours, but not in between," to help eliminate the hunger that promotes binge-ing and provide the necessary structure to contain impulsive eating. Goals are simple and measurable, such as: "Add one slice of cheese to a sandwich at lunch three times this week."

Supervised weighing sessions also give patients opportunities to express their fears and feelings about their weight. Some patients are so terrified of what their weight might actually be that they don't weigh themselves. These fears can be addressed in therapy.

Collaborating with a dietitian

Some therapists collaborate with a trained dietitian to develop nutritious food plans for their patients. These professionals provide an essential link in treatment. Their focus is on designing meal plans that help patients learn to eat normally. Once a patient is better nourished, he experiences fewer emotional upheavals and is able to think about and deal with problems more clearly. The dietitian's training and expertise supports the main idea in the treatment of any eating disorder, which is to separate food- and weight-related behaviors from feelings and psychological issues. In therapy, patients whose eating patterns have been stabilized learn that emotional crises need not trigger episodes of disordered eating.

As we have mentioned previously, the process of treating eating disorders needs to be highly individualized. Again, no single approach to changing behavior works for everyone. Each stage of the process lays the foundation for the next. All change—whether it is psychological, nutritional, or physiological—needs to be gradual. Keep in mind that food control usually creates a critical sense of security for patients and that they are often truly terrified about both losing control and gaining weight.

Challenges to treatment

Even people who truly want to eat normally again and reconnect with their bodies and emotions may have a hard time breaking out of disordered patterns that have become familiar and predictable. However, therapists *can* help patients break through some of the biggest roadblocks to regaining normal patterns of eating and feeling.

Denial

Perhaps the most serious challenge to treatment is denial. If a patient is in such complete denial of his condition that he refuses to participate in treatment, he probably *cannot* be helped unless his condition worsens dramatically. Other levels of denial can interfere with the progress of therapy as well. Here's how they might be overcome:

For people who deny that they have eating and/or body image problems, the therapist might take these actions:

1. Review the foods the patients do or do not allow themselves to eat. Try to get them to acknowledge that they've excluded certain foods and that they have become afraid of a number of foods that they used to enjoy.

2. Discuss ways in which food restrictions limit their social life. For example, they may no longer go out to eat or skip outings because they "feel fat."

3. Discuss the amount of mental energy and time they spend thinking about food and body issues, and describe how this takes away from other areas of their lives.

4. Highlight any moment of misery that they may have acknowledged. Describe how moments such as this one will become more frequent and intense as the disorder grows stronger.

5. Review the physical risks that are inherent in their disordered behavior. If they refuse to pursue psychological treatment, try to get them to have regular medical checkups to ensure their physical health, at the very least. Make the eating disorder into a safety issue.

6. See if they'll agree to nutritional counseling to learn about "safe" foods that can be added to their diet to improve their nutritional health.

7. Describe the sources of eating problems, for instance, that they start from low self-esteem and other stressors. Explain how eating issues become a preferred distraction from relationships, troubled families, difficulties at school, and so on. See if they'll agree to go to therapy to focus on the underlying emotional issues of their disorder.

For people who acknowledge that they have an eating problem but don't want to do anything about it, CBT counselors add a Pros and Cons list to the items listed previously. The list should include secondary gains such as, "I get more attention from friends and family," "It's a good way to get back at people I'm mad at," "It lets me release stress," and so on. If a patient's responses to the list show that the advantages of having a disorder far outnumber the disadvantages, the therapist must then shift the focus away from changing eating patterns to the emotional issues that are highlighted in the list. For example, the therapist might ask the patient what other ways he might get more attention from family and friends, express anger, and release stress. In other words, the focus is now on encouraging the patient to think of more constructive coping strategies.

Personal progress

Many people who have eating problems normalize their behavior and see no need for treatment. Others acknowledge that they might have some "issues" about food and body image, but they feel that their behavior works for them; they feel good about themselves by maintaining this behavior, and they are unwilling to give it up. Still others recognize their disordered behavior for what it is, realize it's *not* good for them, but have strongly ambivalent feelings about giving it up. Even to *attempt* changes in eating, people must have a strong desire to recover from their disorders because the effort required to actually make changes will only increase their anxiety and will make them feel worse before they feel better.

It is essential to work with people at *their* stage of awareness, not to rush to prescribe changes in eating when they're not ready to attempt them. Experienced therapists gear treatment to the ongoing needs of their patients and never force progress where there is too much fear or resistance.

Signs of recovery

While recovery from any eating disorder is a long-term process, there *are* distinct signs of progress. Therapists recognize that a patient is ready to move on when, in addition to stabilizing weight, she demonstrates the following:

- A shift in attitude toward a positive, long view of life

- A breakdown of denial

- Willingness to give up "fear foods" and challenge false beliefs about food

Bright Idea
Therapists sometimes send patients who have difficulty acknowledging the extent of their food restrictions to a grocery store. Each patient is given a list divided into two columns: "Safe Foods" and "Unsafe Foods." As patients go down each aisle and categorize the foods they see, they are often astonished at the number of foods that they have labeled "unsafe" or "forbidden."

A 25-year-old woman who has a long history of Binge Eating Disorder, yo-yoing weight, and constant dieting had 12 weeks of CBT treatment. During this time, she tried to let go of food rules, eat what she wanted, and stop dieting. It was difficult: She was very anxious and experienced a lot of sadness about her slightly overweight body.

A year later, she says CBT changed her life. She now eats whatever she wants, has stopped worrying about food, and has *lost* weight. She has maintained a normal weight for almost a year without dieting or worry, and she says she feels free and grateful.

- The ability to establish flexible, attainable goals that bring success gradually and that aren't focused exclusively on food and body issues

An inside look

People who are engaged in the process of recovery from eating disorders agree that the most important steps to learn are these:

1. How to identify the things that trigger a disorder
2. How to find coping alternatives

For example, fear of school and other social situations may trigger a binge in one patient; among the coping options available to her are learning to talk the fear out or use anxiety-relieving meditation as soon as she feels a twinge of fear. Triggers vary from person to person, as do coping mechanisms. For example, another patient who has anorexia needs to learn to think the rage through and practice more direct and productive ways of expressing her anger, rather than letting it eat at her.

Still, recovery can *feel* uncomfortable, especially when patients are asked to give up familiar patterns of thinking and behaviors that have long served as powerful emotional protectors. To help patients understand and prepare for the difficulties of moving ahead in recovery, therapists discuss *inoculation,* a warning that patients will probably feel worse before feeling better. Therapists sometimes use analogies such as this one to get the point across: "Immediately after surgery, you feel worse than before you went in, but in time, you feel much better." No matter how it is presented, the process of changing eating behaviors undoubtedly increases anxiety and stress. There is simply no way of getting around it. But, as the experts say, the upside is that this anxiety *does* diminish with time.

Side benefits

People in recovery from eating disorders also find other surprising challenges—and rewards. For instance, some patients report that learning to communicate their feelings and express their emotions is not the hardest part of the process: It is *feeling them at all.* At the same time, they discover that the very emotions that they had previously hidden behind food-related behaviors now bring them more satisfaction and enhance their lives in ways they could never have imagined.

This is the kind of shared knowledge that nonprofessional groups can impart as follow-up therapy and that is considered to be a critical part of long-term recovery for many people. Although medical treatment can play an equally valuable role in

❝
Recovery was scary: It was scary to admit to myself that I was in pain, and very scary to relinquish control. But life was better, even during recovery, than it was during the disorder. I discovered that the answers don't have to be scary—instead, they can be care, rest, and food—just the opposite of what I thought I had to put myself through.
—A young man in recovery from an eating disorder
❞

recovery, there is a lot of important information about nonmedical alternatives (see Chapter 12, "Keeping On"). But learning how to select and evaluate professional help comes first.

Just the Facts

- Most eating disorders *can* be treated successfully.

- Successful treatment depends on tailoring tested approaches to individual needs.

- Effective treatment changes a patient's eating patterns, psychological responses, and body perceptions.

- The process may be brief or lengthy, with a single professional or a team, but a careful, step-by-step course can achieve success.

GET THE SCOOP ON...
The choices ▪ Evaluating a
treatment ▪ Networking for information
▪ Covering the costs of therapy

Selecting Treatment

Because both treatments and patients' needs vary so much, it's important to select the most appropriate type of therapy for each individual. A characteristic of many people who have eating disorders is the need for control, so for them it is particularly gratifying to know that there *are* choices to be made on the path to recovery.

Whether you are the patient yourself or someone who is trying to bring a friend or relative who has an eating disorder into treatment, finding the right type of therapy can be the key to successful recovery.

Choosing an approach to therapy

Although there are many specialists who treat eating disorders, some of them focus on only one of the many techniques described in Chapter 10, "The Treatment Process." Some therapists focus only on eating behaviors or emotional issues, while others are more likely to network with dietitians and medicating psychiatrists.

159

Because the patient's full involvement is essential to her recovery, it's important to match treatment with the needs and feelings of the individual whenever possible.

Individual and group approaches to therapy

No single therapeutic approach is exclusively designed to treat eating disorders. As described here, each of them (including 12-step programs) can be practiced in any setting, whether it is a clinic, hospital, residence, or private office.

- Cognitive Behavior Therapy (CBT) stresses changing behavior and learning new patterns of moderating diet. CBT can be done individually or as part of a group. It is practiced by independent therapists or in clinics. Fees vary according to setting.

- The 12-step method is based on abstinence— not eating foods that are troublesome or that may trigger a binge. Overeaters Anonymous (OA) is the most widespread of these. Relying on the shared experience of others who have eating disorders of all kinds, OA requires participa-tion in a group. Group meetings occur daily throughout the country, and participation is free.

- Insight-oriented psychotherapy, which is offered by psychiatrists, psychologists, or social workers, doesn't address eating behaviors at all. Instead, it focuses on issues that underlie eating disorders. Restricting, bingeing, and purging behaviors are seen as symbols of emotional deprivation and unmet needs. Relationships are analyzed to help people discover ways in which their needs are not being met and how to correct this. This form of therapy is usually one-on-one, although it is practiced as a group as well.

- The feminist model of treatment shows women how to overcome conflicting role demands that are imposed on them by society. This model may be at the core of a therapist's approach to treatment, or it can be used in conjunction with other forms of therapy.

- A nutritionist can also provide counseling to people who have eating disorders, either independently or in conjunction with other professionals. Reliable dietitians recognize that treating food-related behavior is not sufficient in itself. Rather, they offer medical nutrition therapy, which, as defined by the American Dietetic Association, is the use of specific nutrition services to treat an illness, injury, or condition. Medical nutrition therapy for eating disorders is a collaborative process in which the registered dietitian and the recovering person work together to change food- and weight-related behaviors. Further psychonutritional therapy entails collaboration with a psychotherapist.

- Group therapy is based on a variety of approaches to treatment; it is led by a professional of one kind or another and meets in sessions. Self-help and mutual-support groups, such as those that follow the 12-step model, are not therapy groups; they are groups that hold meetings.

Because groups offer a variety of approaches to eating disorders—CBT, 12-step, insight-oriented, feminist, or a combination of these—people should find out what exactly is being offered before signing

Bright Idea
When you are
considering a
particular ther-
apy group, ques-
tions such as the
following are
important to
answerbefore
signing up: Is
the group for
people who have
all types of eat-
ing disorders, or
it is just for
those who have
bulimia or
anorexia? What
is the age range?
How many peo-
ple are in it? Is
it a support
group or a ther-
apy group? Is it
structured (that
is, with regular
educational
activities) or
unstructured
(that is, with
people who
speak when they
feel moved to)?
What does it
cost? Can it be
done in conjunc-
tion with indi-
vidual therapy?

up. People who are being treated for eating disorders can participate in both individual and group therapy. For example, issues that are brought up in group therapy can be worked out later, in individual sessions. In a group, people can share experiences and help each other watch for signs of relapse. Participation in a group not only helps members feel less isolated and ashamed, but it also helps them relearn how to see themselves without the distorting filter of their disorder. Twelve-Step and other kinds of support groups offer just that—support—not professional treatment.

Group therapy costs less than individual therapy (sessions average $45 an hour), but there is less individual focus.

Matchups

According to the experts, there really is no best way to match treatments with symptoms. It's really a matter of where the patient feels most comfortable and what seems to work as therapy progresses. CBT, for example, might be the best way to treat binge eating problems and to prepare a patient for later treatment for other underlying conflicts.

A frequently used approach to treatment involves moving patients into insight-oriented psychotherapy once initial food-related behaviors have been balanced by medical, nutritional, and/or behavioral therapy. Insight-oriented psychotherapy helps patients discover new ways to approach relationships without depending on the eating-related structures that once numbed them to emotional issues. This form of therapy also explores and helps to resolve emotional problems that may have created the need for self-starvation. However, the process of coming to terms with food-related issues is ongoing, even as deeper explorations may be taking place. If abuse or other serious dysfunctions have been part of a patient's history, specialized psychotherapy may also be needed at some point.

Evaluating the therapist

Once the patient makes a decision about the best type of therapy, it's important to find the best therapist for him.

The details of a therapist's approach to the treatment of an eating disorder are important, so request specific information at the start.

Just as some treatments for eating disorders are better than others, some therapists are likely to be more effective at treating patients than others. Whether you are considering a psychiatrist, a physician, or a dietitian, what matters the most is proper training. Effective therapy can be provided by almost any type of professional, as long as he or she has the appropriate training and experience.

If you are considering a nutritionist, internist, psychiatrist, or therapist, look for one who specializes in eating disorders. Although all these fields cover eating disorders in their training, generalists often lack the depth of information about treatments that a specialist in eating disorders might have.

Questions to ask

Before you make a decision about using the services of a therapist, make sure that he gives you all the information you need. These are important questions to ask:

- What are your professional credentials?
- Are you a specialist in treating eating disorders?
- What is your approach?

Watch Out!
Some therapists and patients open up deeply traumatic experiences from the past (such as abuse) too early in treatment, and the person's symptoms grow worse. When addressed at a more appropriate time, these kinds of issues can be resolved with fewer symptoms and help the patient grow stronger.

- How long have you been treating patients who have eating disorders, and how many have you treated?

While the specific answers to these questions matter, what is equally important is the way they're answered. Is the therapist willing to answer questions, or is she reluctant? Are his responses thoughtful, or do you sense a hard sell? Beware of any therapist who promises a cure and boasts about his success rate.

People who have been through treatment encourage others to seek help from people and institutions that incorporate a respectful approach to recovery. Therapy is not just about credentials, they say; it's about attitude—the philosophy embraced by a therapist or recovery clinic.

Has the therapist you are considering had any experience with the inner life of people who have eating disorders—with the "voices of anorexia," for instance? Does the therapist seem gentle? respectful? compassionate? Does he seem critical and impatient? Is her approach flexible or rigid? If you don't want CBT, is he willing to try another approach? What type of food program does the recovery clinic or therapist support: abstinence? moderation? force-feeding? What kind of education is provided about nutritional needs? What kind of emotional support is offered? Is family counseling provided? Can the therapist be reached at off-hours?

Asking these questions accomplishes several ends: You will get the information you need to get effective treatment, and the very act of asking questions is important for anyone who needs to take positive control of his or her life. The responses you receive are not only informative; they can tell you a great deal about a therapist. If she does not answer your questions willingly, you have every reason to doubt whether this therapist will be open enough to gain your trust or help you feel comfortable.

Because of the very real fears a patient feels, trust is critical to this relationship. So beware of the therapist who either doesn't return phone calls or who swarms all over you with a sales pitch. Promising too much—guaranteeing a cure, for instance—should make you just as wary as the therapist who seems negative and cold.

Networking

One of the best ways to find an effective therapist is to get information from others who are recovering from eating disorders. You can get referrals from people who have been through it; usually they are quite willing to give evaluations of what their therapy was like.

Just making contact over the telephone with an anonymous person can be difficult enough for someone who has an eating disorder: Isolation is so often a characteristic of the condition, and feelings of shame can make discussion difficult. However, if even a phone call seems overwhelming, your first contact can be with one or more of the organizations that are dedicated to helping people who have eating disorders. These organizations supply educational materials and may provide lists of professionals and free support groups in your area who treat eating disorders. (See Appendix B, "Resource Guide," for more information on these resources, including telephone numbers, addresses, and URLS.)

Rating the resources

Of course, just because information comes from other people who have eating disorders doesn't

Timesaver
While relying solely on the Web is *not* a good idea, it can provide useful background information about how a treatment center or therapeutic group operates before you contact or visit them in person. Use the information you get from the Net as the basis for your own questions.

Tips for Finding a Therapist (in order of effectiveness):

1. Get referrals from others who are in treatment.

2. Call adolescent medicine specialists and see who they recommend.

3. Call your local college counseling center to see if they have an eating disorder specialist on staff or if there is someone in the community to whom they can refer you.

4. Call local teaching hospitals to see if they have eating disorder specialists on staff in their out-patient clinics.

5. Look in the phone book for eating disorder treatment clinics—they are usually found in major metropolitan areas.

6. Check national referral agencies, such as the American Anorexia Bulimia Association (AABA) or other groups listed in Appendix B.

7. Investigate Web sites, but only as a resource or last resort. Practitioners offering treatment via cyberspace cannot really be checked out, and treatment at that distance is not likely to be effective, no matter what the "doctor" promises.

mean it's good—or good for everyone. Questions are in order for even these less formal kinds of treatment as well.

Be aware that a lot of the information available on the Internet is not particularly valuable or even accurate. There are no standards or requirements for publication on the Internet. Anything—whether it is factual or fictional—is publishable. Therefore, beware of anything you read on the Internet. Research into eating disorders is coming up with new causes and solutions at a fairly rapid rate, so "the latest" information is often little better than rumor. Also, myths about eating disorders and their treatment abound. As information spreads on the World Wide Web, it's become clear that misinformation also spreads with lightning speed.

So how can you know what's true? In general, any statement or claim that is extreme, such as, "You will *die* from this disorder!" should cause suspicion. Look for a more measured and reasonable approach, such as: "This is a potentially dangerous disorder that requires treatment to maintain health."

Herbs, acupuncture, or spiritual healing all may indeed have a part in treatment, but relying on a new fad such as the latest in aromatherapy to the exclusion of other treatments is just another form of denial. Turning to a questionable form of treatment can be a way of saying, "My problem is *not* as serious as you say it is. I can manage it with an easy, friendly technique."

The Web itself can be hazardous to recovery as well. While the Internet is great for resources and networking, some sites erroneously claim to provide therapy. Some ask for fees, which can be charged to a credit card. The problem isn't just that there's no way of checking these claims or making a face-to-face evaluation of your own; the real issue is that getting involved with such a nonpersonal form of support is counterproductive because it will not help the person with the eating disorder relearn how to build interpersonal relationships.

Alternative approaches to treating eating disorders may serve as adjuncts to more traditional therapy: Acupuncture, meditation, or herbal therapies, for example, might be of value to some people. In all likelihood, however, these options won't be fully effective by themselves. A better alternative involves starting with traditional therapies and adding alternatives later, if desired. In any case, the therapist should always be aware of other methods used.

How much will it cost?

One reason some people are tempted by spurious offers of cheap and easy treatment is the expense of treating eating disorders legitimately. Indeed, treatment can be costly, but there are ways to make the expense more manageable.

These days one of the most important questions to ask in selecting a therapist or a type of treatment is, "What insurance do you take?" Then ask the insurance company or HMO what treatments for eating disorders they cover—and what their repayment caps are.

Treatment for these disorders can be very costly because, unfortunately, a large number of companies restrict their coverage. Many will not approve coverage unless the patient is seriously suicidal or very close to death. The danger is that the process takes so long that people become dangerously ill before their treatment is financed. By the time admission is approved, the required treatment is much more extensive than it would have been if medical treatment had begun earlier. At this point, a patient is likely to run into an insurance company catch-22: The treatment, which would have been shorter earlier, had it been approved sooner, is now too extensive to be covered.

Some companies consider eating disorders as either a pre-existing condition that their contracts do not cover, or a psychological disorder for which coverage is strictly limited.

Asking questions about money is serious business. A responsible therapist is up front about the costs and will likely use his experience to help find ways to cover costs.

For example, specialists who frequently deal with the hospitalization of people who have eating disorders say that part of the admission process involves getting approval for payment *in advance* from the insurance company. They know that this requires thorough preparation regarding the facts of the case, persistent advocacy, and confirmation of all agreements in writing.

Money matters

Prospective patients should find out *in advance* how much of the total cost of therapy will be covered by their insurance company, HMO, or managed care network.

For example, some insurance companies will pay 80 percent of the fee for a therapist on their list and 50 percent for someone who is not on their list. Find out about annual maximum benefits, that is the maximum number of visits (say, 30 visits a year), or the top dollar amount (perhaps $2,000) per year. You may also want to ask about in-patient mental health benefits:

- Does your policy cover hospitalization? If it does, how many days are covered?

- What is the coverage for hospitals in the network? What about those out of the network?

- Is there coverage for day programs or partial hospitalizations?

Bright Idea
In addition to seeking medical attention and insurance coverage, it is probably wise for patients or their families to employ legal counsel to assure sufficient coverage, especially when the case is serious.

- Is it possible to convert in-patient days to day-program days?

To see someone in your insurance company's network, request their list of eating disorder specialists. Go over the names with your physician or someone in the field who might be able to recommend one. Discuss all the issues, listed above, with your insurance company before you make any decisions. They will give you the information you need to make an evaluation of your options.

Here's another tip that might help bring down the cost of treatment: Find out from your workplace if you can open an account in which to set aside pre-tax money for medical expenses. Many companies permit you to set aside as much as $5,000 per year—before taxes—for anticipated medical expenses. Although this is your own money, avoiding the tax actually increases the amount you have available to spend. Ask your employers if they offer a flexible spending account for medical costs that can save on taxes. Because you pay less tax, it results in a good-sized fund to cover medical costs your insurance company doesn't cover.

Price-conscious treatments

One result of insurance company restrictions is the development of treatments designed to fit within them. For example, even in severe cases of anorexia, short-term intensive care can be provided by less costly treatment at a residential center.

Also, as eating disorders have become more widely acknowledged and accepted as a very serious health concern, a growing number of clinics and counseling centers (especially those in major metropolitan areas and college towns) are providing treatment.

Unofficially...
Seeing a therapist in private practice generally costs between $75 and $125 an hour. A nutritionist can cost about $80 an hour. Psychiatrists usually charge around $150 an hour. Day programs may run to around $350 per day. Some clinics, however, may charge as little as $20 an hour.

Self-help

Serious cases of eating disorders require serious treatment. But self-help can be a beginning, especially if it helps satisfy patients' needs to feel effective and in control. At the very least, self-help can provide an introduction to the kinds of treatments available to people who have eating disorders.

Whether it comes in the form of a book or a Web site, self-help encourages people to go into treatment and offers them the kind of support that groups provide. Self-help systems also have the potential to be a cost-free way of helping some people who might otherwise be afraid to seek treatment. In addition, these systems provide a cost-effective way for clinics to give patients the background they need so that treatment can be made shorter and less costly. Self-help is a beginning, not a cure, but in many cases it provides just the right amount of incentive to move from not doing anything about a serious disorder to thinking seriously about treatment.

Warnings

In the interest of saving money—or out of fear of entering serious treatment—it may be tempting to use less-proven methods of treating eating disorders. Whether they involve the use of prayer or special herbs, these methods may work—but they can also be dangerous if they keep someone from more effective treatments.

Likewise, an individual or organization that offers cheap financing or free consultations should arouse your suspicions—just as it would if someone asked you to sign over all your assets before entering treatment.

Moneysaver
If the cost of therapy is simply too high, or if it is not covered by your insurance, other possibilities include clinics in local teaching hospitals and free-standing clinics that treat eating disorders. Many community mental health clinics have eating disorder specialists and offer sliding-scale fees. The disadvantage of a clinic is that you don't know who you're getting, but the advantage is that it's affordable. If you go to a teaching hospital, in particular, you may even get the benefit of a senior staff member to supervise your treatment.

Watch Out!
People who are
exhausted by an
eating disorder,
or family mem-
bers who are
filled with fear
and guilt may
not use their
best judgment
when it comes
to finding
treatments.
Remember that
the vulnerable
and desperate
tend to be easy
prey for the
unscrupulous.

A positive spin

But it's time to put the negative aside. Here is a story that illustrates the positive results of treatment:

> "It took several attempts before I found doctors who understood what was happening to me and before a diagnosis became clear. An eating disorder recovery specialist, who had experience with cases like mine, and a family practitioner were the two doctors who came up with a diagnosis of depression and an eating disorder. The recovery specialist suggested that perhaps the severity of my ups and downs was chemical, in part, and that drugs might help. She also suggested letting go of my exercise program. What a relief! Little by little I got better, and was able to rebuild my life."

Scary as eating disorders may be, they *are* treatable, and the right treatment does a lot more than simply restore normal eating patterns: It can make life livable again.

Just the Facts

- Almost any school of therapy can treat eating disorders, although most experienced therapists combine knowledge from different schools in order to treat them.

- Training and expertise are critical: Don't be afraid to ask questions before signing on with any therapist.

- Information and support networks are easy to tap into.

- Finding cost-effective therapy is possible with a little investigation.

GET THE SCOOP ON...
Widening the scope of treatment
■ Family and couples therapy ■ Preventing a
relapse ■ Moving ahead

Keeping On

For many people, recovery from an eating disorder is an ongoing process, even if research *has* shown that short-term therapy is highly effective. Still, short or long, recovery is a step-by-step process.

Some people who are in recovery from eating disorders find it helpful to maintain an awareness of their former condition to avoid relapse. Others who are sensitive to the onset of a disorder have a plan in place to contact a therapist or support group to nip an episode in the bud. Or, through treatment, some people become aware of the events or emotional situations that are most likely to trigger old behaviors. Taking extra care to eat regularly and touch base with a counselor keeps others from overreacting to old but distinctly dangerous triggers.

A recovery-support network can be invaluable in preventing relapse, but even a surprisingly simple activity such as keeping a journal can increase a person's awareness of potentially dangerous patterns.

Both patients and therapists note that the wider and deeper the therapy—including family therapy,

Chapter 12

66

I am at a stage now where I never dreamed I would be. Overcoming the demons that fuel an eating disorder is hard, very hard. But it is possible! With the proper professional therapy and a great support system outside therapy, it is amazing what can happen: Sitting down to a meal and enjoying every forkful, for instance, is an amazing experience in itself.
—A young man, in recovery from anorexia

99

support group activity, and perhaps in-depth psychotherapy or even spiritual realignment—the greater the benefits. When both eating and emotional issues are addressed, the longer lasting and more effective the recovery, and the greater the preparedness to avoid relapse.

Expanding the goals of recovery

"Getting better" from an eating disorder means more than simply attaining a balanced weight or being free of such symptoms as purging or bingeing. Recovery means going on to a normal and comfortable life.

Getting back to "normal"

For people who have eating disorders, part of getting better and being "normal" is learning how to be comfortable in social eating situations. In fact, one indication of recovery is being able to eat with people in a normal fashion. Typically, these individuals are most likely to have stayed away from social eating during their illness—or perhaps they may always have had profound social difficulties that were masked by an eating disorder of one kind or another.

Support groups and family counseling can help with this important aspect of ongoing recovery. Like most aspects of recovery from an eating disorder, socializing may take time and patience. However, it's a very important sign of health.

Exercise, too, is a "normal" part of life. But for people in treatment for eating disorders, adding exercise must be done carefully because overexercise may be part of their disorder. Of course, exercise can contribute a sense of well-being and bring body functions into balance, but it must be monitored. Family and friends also need to understand that even former patients shouldn't be urged to join in a bike-hike right away.

Likewise, people who are recovering from eating disorders are advised to move gradually back into normal work patterns and social activities—especially if they had had a previous tendency to do all things "perfectly."

In sum, learning to bring moderation into every aspect of life is an important factor in long-term recovery. To live consciously with this kind of balance (something that many of us strive for) is one of the unexpected benefits of recovering from an eating disorder.

There are many ways of encouraging this kind of wider recovery. The next sections examine some of these.

Family therapy

Family therapy entails a wide range of techniques and approaches, depending on the needs of the person who is in recovery from an eating disorder. For example, some adults who are trying to separate from their families may not want them involved. Others, however, may want help in negotiating support from family members, and request that they be involved in treatment. The goals of family therapy can be as far reaching as a total restructuring of the family itself.

Family or marital counseling may be valuable if depression or substance abuse is present in the family. At the very least, family therapy calls for counseling by the staff of an eating disorders clinic or the patient's therapist. In these cases, even a simple, limited goal, such as the support of the person who has the disorder, is important. Some families choose to find therapy for themselves, regardless of

Unofficially...
According to the American Dietetic Association, the name "eating disorder" is somewhat misleading because it implies that the essence of the problem is disordered eating and that the solution is learning to eat normally again. However, changes in eating and related behavior may not be enough. Changes in relationship patterns may also be crucial for the person to be nourished emotionally, as well as physically.

Watch Out!
When the mother of a patient who has bulimia and who is unable to stop purging called her daughter's therapist to ask if she should try "tough love" (that is, getting angry at her daughter), she learned that this was *not* an effective strategy. Gentleness is more appropriate.

whether the person in their family who actually has the eating disorder chooses to do so.

For children and adolescents living at home, family therapy is an important component of treatment because it helps give them a broader understanding of eating disorders. At the same time, it gives families the tools to manage difficult feelings, such as anger and guilt, which are often directed toward the person in the family with the eating disorder. Clearing away some of those tensions and conflicts can sometimes improve relationships within the family in general.

Adults who don't live with their families may not want or need family therapy. However, they may want individual family members to come with them for one or two sessions to address a single issue or receive more general information about a disorder. Sometimes this form of participation and interest fosters the growth of new emotional connections within a family.

Couples therapy is for people living with a spouse or a partner. Issues such as the ones noted for the family are addressed here as well. For example, a woman who has bulimia may get angry at her husband for any number of reasons, but instead of addressing him directly with her grievances, she may binge and purge to relieve herself of her anger. Learning to address conflicts more directly within her marriage through couple's therapy may relieve her symptoms and have even wider beneficial effects for the relationship.

Family therapy can be quite significant for long-term, in-depth recovery. The same suggestions that apply to choosing therapy for an individual patient apply to choosing family therapy. In some cases, however, the same therapist who treats the patient treats the family as well, unless the situation is quite complex.

Relapse prevention

Families worry about their loved one having a relapse. Relapse also is a huge concern for patients themselves, especially for those who have struggled with relapse on more than one occasion. The good news is that there *are* techniques to help avoid relapse.

Relapse prevention simply means taking the time with the patient to do the following:

- Review strategies that have proven helpful in controlling symptoms

- Identify steps to take during stressful times, when a relapse may occur

- Educate the patient about lapses (they're not the same as a relapse), normal bingeing, signs of trouble, and triggers to catch in order to prevent an relapse

These are some of the steps a therapist takes to keep a patient safe from the dangers of relapse:

1. Reminding the patient that a *lapse* (that is, a temporary regression to old patterns) does not mean a relapse. It is simply a temporary setback that can be easily corrected and from which one can learn a great deal. A *relapse*, on the other hand, requires help from a professional.

2. Reminding the patient that sometimes most people eat more than they think they should. This is not abnormal, nor is it a sign of loss of control.

3. Considering which elements of the patient's treatment were found to be most helpful.

Unofficially...
According to the American Dietetic Association, eating disorders are complex illnesses that involve two sets of issues and behaviors: those directly relating to food and weight, and those involving relationships with oneself and others.

Preparing a written plan for the patient helps her manage eating when it becomes a problem.

4. Reminding the patient to expect occasional setbacks, and encouraging him to utilize the skills he has learned to deal with eating problems as they arise.

5. Stressing (again) the risks of dieting. The therapist explains that the patient may be tempted to diet in the future, but she must have serious reservations about doing so.

6. Discussing legitimate reasons for dieting, such as if the patient is clearly overweight, compared to his own norm, or if the patient needs to lose weight for medical reasons.

Taking life easy

People who are close to someone who has been treated for an eating disorder also need to be aware of the steps that prevent relapse. A feeling of always being watched by family and friends, however, does not contribute to a contented, useful, and relapse-free life; the more relaxed everyone is, the more comfortable things will be for the whole family.

To achieve a relaxed and rewarding life after treatment, some people find it valuable to stay in touch with the process of recovery by joining a chat room on the Web or by touching base with a support group periodically. Reaching out to help others who are struggling with a disorder can help strengthen one's own recovery.

On the other hand, some people in recovery no longer want to associate with people who have eating disorders because they feel guilty, envious, or competitive with them. Other people simply prefer to forget the period in their lives when they had a disorder and want to spend time with people who don't focus on illness. Therefore, they put their energy into moving ahead with their lives and let newfound successes replace the food obsessions of the past.

Steps ahead

Having moved away from the scariest, most active aspects of recovery, many people find ways to benefit by viewing recovery as a positive growth experience.

Journaling is one technique used to explore other aspects of recovery. Some people find that keeping a journal is a good way to cope with the daily stresses of life that might otherwise activate a relapse. Keeping a journal is also a good way to express emotions, especially for those who find the process difficult. Other forms of creative expression—in art or music, for instance—offer similar outlets and sources of inspiration for people who are in recovery.

What it feels like

People who have gone through treatment for eating disorders say: "It is a lot of work, but you learn that you are a great person and that nothing or no one can make you feel less than anyone else. You'll learn to ditch your own rules and make new ones to get what you truly deserve."

Others report this kind of accomplishment, which is never easy: "Some of what I dealt with was very scary and also exciting: showing emotions! My goal is to get angry without being afraid that I'm going to hurt someone, to cry without thinking that I'm ugly."

Although it is important to be optimistic about recovery, it helps to know that the process doesn't necessarily have a distinct beginning or end; like anything else in life it is part of an ongoing process.

> "
> Overcoming my eating disorder was the hardest thing I've ever had to do, but it was well worth the effort. I even moved beyond getting better. I feel strong and proud of my accomplishment. I learned so much about myself and my family. I sought and received help from friends who also had eating disorders, and I helped my dad, who, like me, suffered from depression. When I was going through therapy, I felt as though I had wasted part of my life. Now I know that all those years of suffering have made me who I am. They made me strong, and they gave me a purpose. I wouldn't go back and change a single day of my life, but I wouldn't spend another second starving myself, either.
> —A young woman in recovery
> "

As one recovering patient put it, "Getting better has been one of the hardest but also one of the most rewarding achievements of my life. However, I still have a long way to go in recovery—and in learning how to cope with the next thing life throws at me."

Beyond coping

"Getting better," of course, means a lot more than "not relapsing." It's about living. People who have been through the process provide these reminders of how to go about getting a life:

- Practice self-affirmation. Every day, tell yourself out loud: "I deserve to enjoy my life!" This will help give you a positive mind set and begin to correct the negative self-talk that is so common in people who have eating disorders. Although you won't necessarily believe the messages you're trying to send to yourself, they can stand as a correction to negative self-statements. Once you begin to detach from them, you will be able to move on to more positive feelings and thoughts about yourself.

- Find what works for you. Is that painting? School? Singing, reading, or writing? Support groups or spirituality? A new career or an old fishing pole? Go for the joy.

- Take a class in something you've always wanted to do. Learn to play a musical instrument, begin writing in a journal every day, or find a friend and go to a movie.

- Don't be afraid to say no to people or to say yes to something totally new.

Just the Facts

- Treatment for eating disorders means much more than restoring normal eating patterns.

- Families and patients alike can receive unexpected benefits from therapy.

- A relapse isn't necessarily a bad thing; it can provide a valuable learning experience.

- Letting go of an eating disorder leaves emotional room for other, more rewarding activities.

Living with Someone Who Has an Eating Disorder

PART V

GET THE SCOOP ON...
Getting some distance ▪ Taking practical
steps ▪ Managing daily life ▪ Handling a relapse
▪ Learning from the experience

How to Help Someone You Love

Chapter 13

As complex as it is for people to cope with and recover from eating disorders, their experiences can also send shock waves through the lives of their families and friends.

For anyone who is close to someone who has an eating disorder, this chapter offers guidelines on how to help. Chapter 14, "Helping Yourself," covers the equally important topic of how to find help for yourself.

In every life crisis or trauma, there are primary victims and indirect victims. People who are struggling with eating disorders are suffering directly, while those around them suffer indirectly. But no matter how you cut it, everybody hurts.

Separating feelings from facts

The process of coming to terms with a loved one's eating disorder consists of three stages:

1. Developing awareness of the scope of the problem

2. Adapting one's attitude toward it and

3. Taking actions that actually help

Here, "awareness" is not about suspicions of an eating disorder, as it was in Chapter 9, "What to Do If Someone You Know Has an Eating Disorder," but about what eating disorders look like and how to approach the people who suffer from them. For the indirect victims—the people who are close to someone who has an eating disorder—awareness of their own "condition" is equally important. In other words, the parent, spouse, sibling, or friend of someone who has an eating disorder is likely to experience fear, guilt, anger, and grief.

It's important to acknowledge these feelings and deal with them directly because they can lead to frustrating and futile attitudes and actions that range from deep denial to obsessive efforts to control the person with the eating disorder. Neither approach works very well. Instead, it takes a change of attitude that balances acceptance of the situation with a willingness to take actions that actually help.

It can be excruciatingly painful to be close to someone in the throes of an eating disorder, but it's important to separate one's own feelings from the facts of the disorder itself. In other words, it helps enormously to look at the eating disorder as the culprit, not the person who is suffering from it. Suspending judgment is essential; it is pointless to blame anyone for an eating disorder. Recovery should always be the main goal.

Taking action

The first step toward helping someone who has an eating disorder is gaining an understanding of what can and cannot be done.

Learning as much as possible—getting all the facts—about a disorder from books like this one can be very useful. (For other sources, see Appendix B, "Resource Guide.") Knowledge can lead to a better understanding, for example, of what lies beneath certain behaviors—especially the frightening ones—that are very often associated with eating disorders. It is a tremendous relief to know that these behaviors stem from the victims' inner conflicts and that they do not represent willful attacks on the people who love them.

Gaining a more personal, firsthand understanding of an eating disorder is just as valuable. Loved ones should visit a few support groups for people who have eating disorders, either alone or with the person with the eating disorder. Or, they might spend some time visiting various Web sites and chat rooms to get a better sense of what the disorders are all about.

Without both factual and firsthand knowledge, it is difficult to understand these irrational disorders, especially when so many misconceptions about them exist. For example, the idea that eating disorders are just about "eating," or that disordered behavior is within the control of its victims, is simply not true—yet these ideas persist.

Calming down

But sometimes knowledge is not enough. For one thing, just knowing about eating disorders will not help your loved one let go of his, nor will it give you the power to control his behavior. What is needed is a profound change in attitude.

First of all, intense emotional responses to life-threatening illnesses such as anorexia and bulimia need to be modified. For example, parents very

> 66
> Anorexia not only destroys the lives of its victims, but those who love and care for them as well. My husband felt helpless throughout my illness. It tore him apart.
> —A wife and mother in recovery
> 99

❝
Our daughter just happens to have a disorder called anorexia and sees no hope right now. So I say there is hope... and I pray... or just listen. I want to reach into her spirit and remove the pain and darkness.
—A mother
❞

Bright Idea
List some things about your own life that you can change. List some things about your loved one's life that you *can't* change. Decide to focus on the things you can change.

often react to feelings of helplessness with guilt, terror, and despair; or they rage over behavior that seems so simple to fix: "If only she would just eat! But instead, she makes everyone around her miserable!" These reactions are understandable, but to be really helpful, loved ones need to get past them and truly accept the situation.

Telling someone who has anorexia or bulimia that she is "willful" or "selfish" will only backfire and reinforce the negative views of herself that this person already has. Understand that what most of us perceive as obstinacy in a person who has anorexia is in reality an outgrowth of her terror of gaining weight. And blaming her for "failing" to seek treatment will only worsen her feelings of shame and guilt.

Understanding that your loved one is not doing anything *to* you also is critical: "If she can't help herself and won't let others help her, why does she hurt me so much?" a parent asks. What this parent needs to remember is that her daughter is not *trying* to hurt her; in fact, she can't help what she's doing.

First steps

An eating disorder may be clear to everyone but the person who has it. Rather than tell that person that he has bulimia or anorexia, it's better to help him discover it for himself. Gently introduce him to the possibility by asking him to consider the questionnaire on the following page:

What to do over the long run

Staying calm and upbeat is important because victims of eating disorders need to be treated gently, patiently, and with a positive attitude. In fact, working to maintain this kind of attitude is an important action in itself, one that can help lessen feelings of

Do You Have an Eating Disorder?

Check out your own susceptibility to an eating disorder. Answer "yes" or "no" to each of the following questions:

- Have you ever fasted to lose weight?
- Do you feel guilty when you eat?
- Do you ever vomit, take laxatives, or use diuretics to control your weight?
- Does your daily weight determine how happy you are for that day?
- Do you feel fat even though people say you're thin?
- Have you ever sneaked or stolen food, diet pills, or laxatives?
- Do you collect lots of recipes?
- Do you carefully count calories?
- Do you go on regular eating binges?
- Are you afraid of losing control?
- Do you feel you'll never be good enough?
- Do you follow any eating rituals?
- If you break your eating or exercise patterns, do you feel guilty or frightened?
- Do you exercise more than one hour every day?
- Do you lie about how much you eat or don't eat?
- Do you have irregular menstrual periods?

If you answered "yes" to three or more of these questions, you may be at risk for a serious health problem. Talk to your family, partner, doctor, therapist, or a good friend about it. Help is available.

despair and helplessness. What is not required is smothering or caretaking. Instead, matter-of-factly accept the realities of the situation and move as calmly and thoughtfully as possible toward maintaining a hopeful and helpful environment.

Just for parents

When you are the parent of a child or a teenager who has an eating disorder you can't simply switch off your emotions, of course. It's your job to keep your child safe and healthy, so you must seek treatment for her.

Still, the disorder and the child must be handled with respect and with the realization that she is not doing anything on purpose TO you.

The box on the following page, "Tips for Parents," offers some guidelines that may help if a parent suspects that a child's eating habits are disordered.

Managing daily life

Getting through a day—or just a meal—without painful conflicts over food-related behavior is a great achievement. The right kind of communication can also aid recovery. Here are some tips:

- Let your child be in charge of what he eats, unless his therapist has advised otherwise.

- Don't monitor how much or how little food is eaten. Eating and weight are *only part* of an eating disorder. If weight drops dangerously, however, consult a doctor right away.

- Always treat your child or teen respectfully and as an equal (unless she is putting herself in real danger).

- Be patient about treatment. There is no magic cure.

Tips for Parents

Although it's true that children who have eating disorders need guidance from their parents, they should be allowed a measure of control over their own lives as well.

Express compassion and concern toward your child, but not anger; be as matter-of-fact as possible about his behavior.

Avoid focusing on your child's "looks." Comments such as, "You're looking far too thin," or "You're looking great!" (if your child is very thin) don't help. Both approaches encourage children to be overly self-conscious about their bodies.

Explain what you suspect by detailing behaviors. Observations should be stated using "I" phrases, such as: "I'm noticing that you are skipping meals and eating less. I am concerned for your health."

Discuss your concerns with your child's pediatrician, if she is still a minor. Take your child to the doctor for checkups and for treatment of any of the *side effects* of an eating disorder, even if your child is unwilling to accept that he has a disorder.

As your child begins treatment, be caring, but do not discuss eating, weight, or appearance. Likewise, do not insist that your child eat or change behaviors.

Finally, be willing to work with your child's therapist and consider finding help for yourself as well.

- Keep in touch with your child's therapist or team of therapists. Although it's not a good idea to interfere with treatment, it is worthwhile to request re-evaluation if you haven't seen any results over the course of a few months. Parents have rights, of course, but therapists have more experience with treating eating disorders; it is generally more effective to follow their advice and suggestions.

- Again, do your best to avoid commenting on your child's appearance or behavior. If you are concerned, discuss the matter with your child's therapist.

- Remember that even the people you love best (especially your children) may get angry and upset with you, despite the fact that you are only trying to help. Keep in mind that the child who has a disorder is frightened and feels the need to defend it. Fighting only makes his fear worse.

Managing mealtimes

Understandably, mealtimes can be the source of a great deal of tension if you live with someone who has an eating disorder. Try these suggestions for getting through them as smoothly as possible:

- Do have regular family mealtimes. Dinner together isn't always possible, but try to maintain a regular schedule of family meals, and ask the person who has an eating disorder to show up for it. He will be more likely to come if the scene at the table isn't unpleasant. Don't make it into a big deal!

- Don't change family patterns to accommodate an eating disorder. For example, continue to prepare normal foods. If you start planning menus around a person who has anorexia, for

example, no one wins because you can never—
or very rarely—please her. Some families twist
themselves into pretzels trying to fulfill the
impossible demands of an eating disorder. This
inevitably disrupts family life and breeds resentment and frustration.

- Don't talk about food at the meal. For example,
  don't say, "Wouldn't you like some of this?
  There's no fat in it."

- Avoid watching or staring at the person while
  he eats.

- Try to keep the conversation light and focused
  on things besides food, weight, eating disorders,
  and so forth. Incorporate all family members
  into the conversation; for instance, be sure that
  siblings have the opportunity to talk about what
  they did that day.

- If you notice problems, such as the person playing with food, spitting into a napkin, or eating
  less and less, bring your concerns to the therapist rather than becoming the "food police."

Bottom-line protections

Family members may not be able to cure or control
the behavior associated with an eating disorder, but
they can do things to ease its course and protect a
child, spouse, or partner from some of the worst
damage it can do. One way of accomplishing this
may be to say, "I understand that you don't want to
eat, but I would feel better if you tried to drink a
little water or helped yourself to one of the liquid
meals or nutrition bars I've left in the kitchen cabi-
net." Say that it will make *you* feel better and that
you are not trying to interfere. Work with the therapist to encourage intake of liquids and food.

Watch Out!
Beware of
becoming the
"food police."
Being too watch-
ful about food
intake and mak-
ing suggestions
about eating are
steps that go
over the line and
may backfire,
causing both the
sufferer and her
family to feel
worse.

Because over-the-counter digestive aids (such as Maalox) can help counter the effects of purging, families may want to keep supplies of these on hand.

It might seem that following these suggestions is the equivalent of giving in to an eating disorder or enabling the sufferer to continue a pattern of illness. On the contrary, delicately helping a person to cope *does* protect his health—albeit to a limited degree—and may be a step toward gaining trust.

More matter-of-factness

Although the calm day-to-day acceptance of an eating disorder can smooth the experience of living with someone who has one, it doesn't mean that you are ignoring the situation or that you need to keep pretending it's not there.

You can be open and honest about the facts of an eating disorder while assuring the person of your emotional, practical, and, if appropriate, financial support. At the same time, keep these tips in mind:

- Continue to communicate your concern and the belief that treatment is necessary.

- Don't get involved in discussions about an eating disorder unless you are knowledgeable about treatments and know which ones to suggest.

- Take responsibility for getting minors into treatment. If your child is under the legal age of adulthood in your state, you as a parent have the right and the responsibility to see that she gets medical help.

- Express your understanding and willingness to participate in and support complex treatment that involves the physical, psychological, and behavioral aspects of the disorder, both for the child and the family.

- Be as supportive and understanding as humanly possible, but don't allow the direct victim to disrupt your own life with manipulative and potentially hazardous behavior, whether it is intentional or not. Be willing to participate in family therapy. Consider patterns of your own that might contribute to the disorder, and be open to hearing the person's perceptions of you and your relationship with her.

In case of relapse

Recovery from an eating disorder does not usually follow a straight, steady line. Most people *do* recover, but it can be a long process, even after initial therapy is completed. Recovery also requires the patience and tolerance of all concerned.

This does not mean constantly monitoring the person with the disorder—that's likely to backfire. Quietly staying alert to signs of relapse, however, can prove valuable, especially because the sufferer may not be able or willing to admit that it's happening.

One of the most obvious things to do is to look for signs that the person is becoming more obsessive about food and weight. For instance, is she

- Weighing herself often, eating ritualistically, or looking in the mirror frequently?
- Expressing perfectionist attitudes?
- Expressing feelings of hopelessness?
- Isolating and withdrawing herself?
- Eating more diet foods or overexercising?
- Wearing only loose-fitting clothes?

These can be signs of a relapse that warrant caring comments and very gentle probing.

Moneysaver
If the therapist who is oversee-ing your child's treatment sug-gests that family members attend sessions, accept the offer. Resisting may not only be counterproduc-tive and prolong therapy, but it also may cost more over the long run.

What is gained

People do get to the other side of eating disorders, but it can be difficult for family members to make the adjustment. Therapists say that it's as important for those who are close to people in recovery to let go of the disorder as it is for the recovering person.

"First, you have to think 'disorder' and get used to that. Then, you have to learn to think 'health' and move on," one doctor puts it. This doesn't mean sweeping the disorder under the rug and pretending it never happened, but it does mean assuming a more positive attitude in general. The assumption should be that all will be well. Family members also should try to relax and stop watching so intensely for the disorder to reappear.

One thing that can help is to do a little soul-searching to discover what coping with an eating disorder has done for the family: "What have I learned from this? How has this trouble strengthened my family and me and enhanced our lives?"

With this kind of positive attitude, families can move on a little more easily.

What recovery feels like

No matter how practical and accepting family and friends are about handling the eating disorder of someone who is close to them, the pain is very real nevertheless. Insights into this can be gained from the stories and comments of others who have gone through the experience.

For example, one parent writes: "It is a living hell, for you and your child. But remember that you cannot cure him; he has to want to get well. Give him your love and support, but also take care of yourself. Just hug your child and let him know you love him. Most children want to get well, but it takes a long time."

A father describes watching the progress of his daughter's eating disorder:

> "As early as 14 or maybe 13 years of age, she began to seek 'control' of her life by not eating. By the time she was 17, she had built a wall around herself that no one could penetrate, not her family… not her friends. There was such a wild mixture of emotions… intense feelings inside me, her dad. There was sadness, anger, frustration, and an indescribably deep, deep hurt because under it all, I *loved* that little girl. Her siblings (two sisters and two brothers) and my wife could not understand why she repelled and pushed them away when all they wanted to do was love her. We all felt guilty and hurt together."

Living with that kind of hurt can make it very hard to provide the kind of careful, just-right help that someone who has an eating disorder needs. That's one reason why families and friends may need support for themselves, as we discuss in Chapter 14 "Helping Yourself."

Just the Facts

- The pain of living with or being close to someone who has an eating disorder is real.

- You can take steps to ameliorate the physical and emotional effects of living with someone who has an eating disorder.

- Family and friends can be supportive without giving in or pandering to an eating disorder.

- Staying calm and learning what you can about the disorder, the victim, and yourself are the keys to assisting recovery.

GET THE SCOOP ON...
Why you need help ▪ Finding family
support ▪ Seeking professional therapy
▪ Using support networks

Helping Yourself

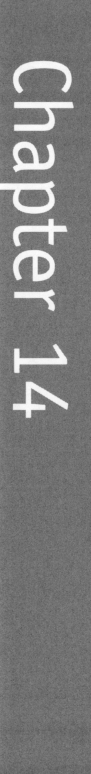

You can see what anorexia is doing to your daughter—but can you see what it's doing to you? Unfortunately, some families can't see: The power of denial can be as strong in the people who are close to someone who is suffering from an eating disorder as it is in the sufferer herself. In fact, denial can be so strong—especially when it is compounded with other powerful emotions—that it eats away at the lives and stability of loved ones.

Many families refuse to consider help for themselves because their guilt over what they perceive as their "failure" is so strong. But families need to realize that if they can find help for themselves, they'll be much better equipped to help the ones they love.

Some families feel they can tough it out and let the person in their family who has the eating disorder cope with it on he's own, while at the same time insisting that they're "fine." Unfortunately, this kind of attitude masking as tough love causes emotional trouble sooner or later.

Unofficially...
One of the most difficult aspects of struggling with another's eating disorder is feeling so alone. Yet for each case of an eating disorder, there are usually more than a few friends and relatives who share the same feelings and experiences.

This chapter focuses on what families and friends can do to save themselves from the damaging ripple effects of an eating disorder.

Why you need help

Whatever the disorder, the caretakers of the people who suffer from it experience deleterious effects themselves. This psychological truth has become so well accepted that publicly funded support—called caretaker relief—is becoming common.

Eating disorders may not be conditions that call for active caretaking by the people around them, at least not at first. But the symptoms of an eating disorder, the fear that surrounds them, and the destructive behavior of those who are afflicted by them can be emotionally and physically draining for the people who live with them. This damage can take several forms, as we'll examine next.

A life of its own

Eating disorders take on a life of their own; people who suffer from them construct rigid systems of living that eventually draw everyone into them unless they are checked. As earlier chapters have shown, the disordered thinking of people whose eating patterns are also disordered can create an almost entirely false view of the world.

Whether trying to cure a disorder or simply adapt to it, families, parents, or spouses sometimes tailor their otherwise normal lives to fit disordered patterns without realizing it. Even people who won't openly admit that their loved one has a problem may be turning their own lives inside out to cope with the situation.

It often takes an outside person—a professional or someone who has shared the same experiences—

Watch Out!
When you find yourself thinking, "I can't sleep at night wondering why this has happened, how she is doing at this moment, and how long will she will live," it is *you* who needs the help.

to see what is happening and to suggest a way to live a healthier life.

Why what you *can't* do can hurt you

In their efforts to cure or control an eating disorder, friends and family sometimes become desperate and depressed. Instead of accepting that they can't cure a disorder, they redouble their efforts and thus increase their feelings of failure.

They may put their own interests and needs aside and focus all their energy on managing the life and health of the person who has an eating disorder. In the process, they effectively let their own lives ebb away, a loss that is unlikely to have any positive effect whatsoever on the life of the person they are trying to help.

Although it is true in most cases that women take on the brunt of caretaking when a family member is afflicted with an eating disorder, and that these responsibilities make it harder for her than for others in the family, men have a hard time, too. If women are pigeonholed as caretakers, men are just as often as not stuck in the role of "fixer" and feel compelled to take charge. It can be difficult to let go of these familiar roles, even when they don't seem to be working particularly well. The truth is that it's hard for anyone to be involved with the care of someone who has an eating disorder. However, for any number of traditional reasons, women are more likely than men to ask for help—either for themselves or for others. Therefore, it is important for men who live with a spouse or partner who has an eating disorder to know that finding good support for themselves will enable them to offer the kind of help that really works.

In other words, letting go and focussing on what they *can* control and manage—their own lives, for

Timesaver
Understanding that you can't cure a person who has an eating disorder saves a lot of time and energy that might better be invested in getting help for yourself.

66

As a man, you're told to do the right thing by providing unconditional love and support, but boy is it difficult.... Men are designed to want to solve problems for others, especially women, whom we feel we should protect. But when all our advice is ignored or rejected, we get resentful, and this frustration is fed right back into the relationship.
—The husband of a woman in treatment after years of bulimia

99

example—ultimately gives caretakers more power to effectively help the person who has an eating disorder.

The family balance

Even under the most optimistic of circumstances—when the direct victim is in treatment and the nature of the condition is in the open, for example—eating disorders can *still* cause terrible imbalances in a family.

A couple may find that the activities they used to enjoy, such as traveling or dining out, are no longer occasions of joy or relaxation anymore because of the extra emotional weight they now carry.

Or, a career may be thrown off track by a spouse's disordered eating patterns and the demands of treatment. Although these dislocations may not seem that serious, they do need attention and discussion before they begin to eat away at a relationship.

In much the same way, the siblings of someone who has an eating disorder may be thrown off balance when so much attention is paid to the primary victim. Depending on their ages and the severity of the situation, their response may be as invisible as low-level resentment, or it may burst into obvious acting out, from trouble in school to overt antisocial activity. Whatever their state of mind, attention must be paid to family members who have had to endure both the illness and the recovery process.

Would therapy help?

For all these reasons, some kind of support for family or friends is extremely valuable. Support may be offered in the simple form of a consultation at a local clinic, or a conversation with a physician or member of the clergy. Brief counseling from an eating disorder specialist can determine very quickly if

Bright Idea
No matter how old they are, the siblings of a person who has an eating disorder need attention, too! Young or grown-up, these people tend to get pushed aside, as so often happens when any kind of family illness occurs. It's very important, therefore, to show them that they are important, too.

more help is needed for all or just some members of the family.

Once the person who has an eating disorder is in treatment, the therapist may want to spend a few sessions talking with other members of the family. It's important to use this opportunity to discuss everyone's concerns, not just those of the patient.

Untangling knots

In some cases, the underlying causes of an eating disorder are so complex that family therapy—as well as individual therapy for family members—is recommended. For example, although no firm connection has been established between family psychology and disordered eating, family therapy of some sort may be strongly recommended in some cases where there is a background of family disruption, depression, or child abuse.

Families may strongly resist therapy—after all, it can be extremely painful to look at the past. On the other hand, often the entire family benefits from participation in the treatment of an eating disorder.

Choosing a course for the family

Just as people who have eating disorders have a choice in the type of therapy they prefer, so do their families. Sometimes each parent wants an individual therapist.

Looking at the family as a whole, family therapy usually tries to take the focus off the sick child to explore how other family members may be helping to create imbalances and dysfunction.

While families may benefit from counseling or support, it doesn't necessarily mean a commitment to long-term, in-depth psychotherapy. In fact, it can boil down to a few conversations. In any case, it is very beneficial to participate, not only for the sake

Unofficially...
Therapy for eating disorders can throw off a family's balance just as effectively as the eating disorder itself can. Unhealthy patterns that build up around a disorder need to be changed as treatment begins to restore health not only to the primary victim, but also to her family.

of the victim, but also for the entire family. So, when a therapist or clinic recommends family involvement, take the opportunity.

Nonprofessional support groups also exist for families. The difference between these groups and professional counselors is that they are free. Another difference is that professionals in the treatment of eating disorders usually focus on how family and friends can help the patient rather than on how they can help themselves. Naturally, these therapists also have an interest in helping indirect victims find their way to health, but this is not their main focus.

Support groups are more likely to focus on how the indirect victims of an eating disorder can manage their *own* lives and detach from sickness to move on, whatever the primary victim's situation. Also, they can provide a network of sources to help inform both patient and family about eating disorders.

Focusing on yourself

To really get help, a family must focus on something other than the person who is ill. For example, the underlying tenets of groups such as Al-Anon, Nar-Anon, or Gam-Anon, where families and friends of various types of addicts find help for themselves, are: "I didn't *cause* the disease, I can't *cure* it, and I can't *control* it." This "three-c" approach can work with families of those who have eating disorders as well.

Some support groups are professionally led, others are therapy groups moderated by a therapist, and some are nonprofessional self-help organizations whose members share their own experiences without offering professional advice.

Letting go

For the family of someone who has an eating disorder, one of the hardest things to do is let go. The

Timesaver
If you can't find a support group for families of people who have eating disorders nearby, sit in on a few Al-Anon meetings, which come together regularly in most communities around the country. You may find valuable ideas there for living your own life while "detaching with love" from the person in your life who has an eating disorder.

reason for this is that overcontrol, to the point of smothering, is a common characteristic of families that foster eating disorders—whether they intend to or not. Therapists have observed that one unconscious motive for rigidly controlled eating in people who have eating disorders characterizes the person who is in need of standing up for herself and being heard.

Just as professionals advise the person who has an eating disorder to make her own decisions, members of support groups, people who have been through the experience themselves, tell family members that letting go is the key to moving on. Letting go is not the same as pushing away the person who has the disorder; rather, it means releasing the hold that the disorder has on the family.

Letting go also involves acceptance that one can only do so much to help the victim: It's possible to care about him without taking care of her. And this offers the freedom to let a loved one find her own way.

What's on the Web?

Take a look at the lists of organizations in Appendix B, "Resource Guide,"—any of them offers help in finding professional and nonprofessional support related to eating disorders.

A vast number of Web sites are related to eating disorders on the Internet. The quality of the information varies, but it can point you to organizations that offer support nevertheless. At many sites, the stories and personal experiences provide a real sense of support for anyone who is struggling with a disorder, whether it is their own or someone else's. But it is wise not to sign on and get too involved: At these sites and throughout the Web, you don't know

Watch Out!
The Web can provide a valuable network of information—and it's best to explore it just for that rather than get enmeshed personally with anyone you meet there. If you do connect with someone on the Web, do it anonymously. Remember that you may be emotionally vulnerable and thus open to misuse by someone who is less than healthy.

who's actually on the other end of the wire. Still, sharing the experience of struggling with an eating disorder with someone "nearby" can give you the feeling of not being quite so alone.

For example, the sister of a young woman who died of an eating disorder started a Web site that not only helps ease her pain, but it also gives support to others who are going through the same anguish. At another site, a father describes his journey through his daughter's eating disorder and gets relief while sharing his strength and experience. You can do the same because Web sites and home pages are easy to set up. But again, caution is in order: Unfortunately, the vulnerability you reveal may attract interest and contact from people whose intentions are not sincere. Be careful. Some people use the Web to exploit and manipulate others, whether they are conscious of it or not.

Perhaps the most useful service offered by Web sites is to help people see the value in finding support and to point them toward sources closer than cyberspace.

From the inside

These stories from people who are close to someone who has an eating disorder are fairly typical of the personal experiences you'll find on the Web:

> A 21-year-old college student in New York has a girlfriend who has been suffering from anorexia for almost eight years. She was doing okay at school, he says, but over the summer break she has relapsed. A lot of her friends have given up on her; for the most part, her family has, too. But he refuses to give up, he says, because he can tell when her disease is talking and when *she* is. He says that

he "really hates this thing that is trying to kill her," but he tries to deal with it by separating her from the disease—and he loves her all the more.

A woman whose sister has been struggling with anorexia for over three years talks about going through the agony of watching her deteriorate, despite hospitalization and counseling. She understands that there's a "monster" in her sister's mind and despairs of ever seeing her recover. At the same time, she also admits that she is in pain herself, from being forgotten about and put aside while everyone—especially family and friends—pour their time and attention into caring for and worrying about the person who has the disorder. "Siblings," she says, "experience pain waiting for recovery."

These very personal stories from the Web give an idea of the kinds of struggles people endure and have the strength to share. But help *is* available, as this chapter has shown.

While it is true that an eating disorder can harm not only the victim but also those around her, it is also true that an eating disorder can be a trigger to motivate a family or an individual to find. Benefits *can* be gained, whether the disorder itself is cured or not.

Just the Facts

- Getting help for yourself can help the sufferer—and make your own life more worthwhile, too.

- Whether families are asked to come into the therapeutic process or not, they may benefit from getting help themselves.

- Families and friends have a variety of choices for support and treatment.
- Used wisely, the Web can be a good resource, if only to demonstrate that you are not alone in the struggle.

GET THE SCOOP ON...
What parents can do ▪ Making food messages
positive ▪ Healthy rules ▪ Lightening up

How to Prevent Eating Disorders

The best way to treat eating disorders—and relapses as well—is to prevent them. So whether you are a parent or another family member who is interested in avoiding disordered eating in children, or a survivor of an eating disorder yourself, there are a number of ways to stay on the healthy side of food.

The parent factor

As discussed in Chapter 1, "Food, Body Image, and Self-Esteem," parental influences on disordered eating patterns are sometimes deep-rooted and complex. Therefore, it's important to look at these roots first. We'll also explore how parents and families can help change attitudes about food, defuse harmful media messages, and most importantly, prevent children from using food as a means of emotional expression.

Strong evidence indicates that distorted body perceptions underlie eating disorders. Therefore,

Unofficially...
According to
The American
Dietetic Associa-
tion, there is no
better time than
childhood to
make an impact
on the lifelong
eating and exer-
cise habits that
contribute to
health mainte-
nance and dis-
ease prevention.

learning to feel comfortable with one's body will obviously help avoid the development of an eating disorder. Of course, there is no single, magical solution to the complexities of an eating disorder, and prevention cannot be reduced to following a few simple steps.

However, it does help to focus on a few relatively straightforward methods of prevention. If research has shown that dieting triggers eating disorders, it makes sense to stop dieting. This cannot be accomplished in a vacuum, though, so parents need to counter their children's overconcern with dieting and body shape. One way is to help them look under their skin and beyond appearance to discover real, personal value. Essentially, the goal is to allow food and the way we judge our bodies to be *only* a part of our lives instead of a reason for living. This also involves making the activities that should be fun— eating and playing, for example—instead of competitive and all-important. This chapter makes a few suggestions that might ease the way.

Changing the message

Often without realizing it, and with the best of intentions, parents and other adults send body image messages to children very early on in life: They tell toddlers how "cute" their "little" bodies are, and the media (especially television) constantly bombards the youngest watchers with messages about diet and body perfection. Although some of these messages get through to children unintentionally, the result is that they *do* learn that "cute" and "pretty" and "slim" are "good."

Children also learn a great deal about cultural attitudes at home. What is a very young girl or boy to make of a mother who doesn't go to the beach because she feels "too fat," or a dad who agrees with her? The lesson, of course, is that "fat" is "bad."

Listening to yourself

With this in mind, parents and other adults should probably spend a little time listening to the kinds of messages they are sending whenever they praise children's bodies. Are you conveying the message that slim is beautiful or that slender is handsome?

Whenever you hear children badmouthing other people for their shape or weight, you can help reverse their attitude by responding honestly with information that conveys a different message. For example you might point out:

> "Some people believe that fat people are bad,
> sick, and out-of-control, while thin people are
> good, healthy, and in-control. This is not
> true, and it's unfair and mean to tease people
> about being too fat, too thin, too short, or
> too tall."

Stereotypes about "fat" people are especially hard to combat because they're so ingrained in our popular culture. But children will undoubtedly feel better about themselves if they receive honest and positive messages about the value and beauty not only of their own bodies, but also of all kinds of body shapes.

Do what I do

Parents also need to look at how they themselves express their own ideas, misconceptions, and stereotypes about diet and body image. For example, are you overemphasizing beauty and body shape, especially with girls?

Make a commitment to help both girls and boys understand the ways in which television, magazines,

Watch Out!
Parental messages about body image, as well as teasing by other family members and peers, have been correlated with body image dissatisfaction and symptoms of eating disorders. Thus parental and peer messages about body shape or weight would seem to exert a strong influence on dissatisfaction with body image.

and other media distort the true diversity of human body types and imply that slender bodies are more exciting, powerful, and beautiful than others.

Be sure to tell even young children that they are growing up just right, and that their bodies are exactly the way they're supposed to be.

Healthier messages

The National Eating Disorders Organization (NEDO) suggests these steps toward helping to prevent the development of eating disorders:

- Build children's self-esteem.

- Accept children regardless of their weight. Let them know that everyone's body is unique and should be valued. Try to model this yourself by accepting your own appearance.

- Teach children to communicate with assertiveness. Children need to be able to resist inappropriate messages from their peers, media, and other adults regarding thinness and self-control over eating and weight.

- Encourage activity and enjoyment of life.

- Do not punish or reward children with food.

- Do not limit caloric intake unless a child's physician requests this due to a medical problem.

- Be open with children. Help them understand the negative consequences of dieting, and help them cope with the pressures of looking a certain way.

- Do not limit your activities because of appearance.

- Eat a well-balanced diet, and set a good example by eating a variety of foods.

Bright Idea
Enlist kids in the anti-diet campaign. Help them counterbalance TV messages with these: If you hear your mom or dad, a sister, or a friend say that someone is too fat and needs to go on a diet, you can say, "I think the person looks just fine the way she is." Or, you can say: "Please don't say that—dieting to lose weight is not healthy, and it's no fun for kids or adults."

Keeping food rules neutral

Of course, families need to have some rules about food so that children develop properly and learn how to feed themselves nutritiously. The message should simply convey that food is meant to be enjoyed and keep people healthy. To accomplish this, children need to eat the foods that will help them grow. It is also very important to emphasize that eating food has nothing to do with being good or bad.

Give kids basic guidelines such as these:

- Eat when you are hungry. Stop eating when you are full.

- Eat a variety of foods—including vegetables and fruits—that you enjoy.

- Eat different types of snacks, too, but if you're bored or sad, try to think of something to do other than eat.

Let kids play with their food and explore all different kinds of tastes, even if they don't eat the whole thing. Let kids "cook" food, too, even if it makes a mess, and close down the Clean-Plate Club for good!

The dinner table is probably the worst place to talk about eating habits. A brief allusion to how much or how little a child is eating might be appropriate, but then the subject should be dropped. Any serious concerns can be raised later.

It's not about food

In the same way that eating disorders are not just about food, as we've discussed earlier, the *causes* of eating disorders are not exclusively about food, either.

For example, people who have problems with disordered eating tend to be perfectionists and are overly demanding of themselves, so these are signs to watch for in children. Parents can help children learn to be more accepting of themselves.

To accomplish this, use praise liberally. It's far better to praise an effort rather than criticize an imperfect result. When a grade comes in lower than expected, ask your child, "How do you feel about that?" rather than berating him; assurance that he'll "do better next time" also is appropriate.

If praise rather than criticism is used, your child will not only be less likely to suffer from eating disorders and other obsessive problems, but she also will be more likely to be creative and easygoing in other aspects of life.

Patterns to watch

Before they are expressed in eating disorders, other patterns of behavior, thoughts, or attitudes may be evident. One of the most potentially damaging attitudes associated with eating disorders—and a real red flag—is perfectionist thinking. For instance, take note if your child's conversation is saturated with "I shoulds" and "I musts." Take care not to express these thoughts yourself. To better assess whether your child is struggling with perfectionist thinking, take a look at the scale on the following page.

If any of these thoughts or beliefs sound as if they might come from your child—or if they sound like something you might say *to* your child, it's a good idea to re-evaluate how you express yourself. At the same time, watch out for signs of eating disorders in a child who seems too "perfect."

Signs of Perfectionism

This inventory lists a number of attitudes and beliefs that sometimes characterize perfectionism:

> If I don't set the highest standards for myself, I am likely to fail.
>
> People will think less of me if I make a mistake.
>
> If I cannot do something really well, there is no point in trying.
>
> I should be upset if I make a mistake.
>
> If I try hard enough, I should be able to excel at anything.
>
> Weakness is shameful.
>
> I shouldn't have to repeat the same mistake many times.
>
> I should scold myself for failing to live up to my expectations.

Good health is a family affair—enjoy it!

While all of us want to be alert to the danger signs of eating disorders, and even though these are viewed as family diseases by some professionals, thankfully there are also positive connections between families and food.

Despite the fact that we are coming to the end of a book about taking eating disorders seriously, an important factor in discouraging these disorders is having fun—enjoying food and establishing pleasurable eating habits. Rather than worrying about body size or monitoring every bite a child takes, parents need to adjust their own attitudes first to show their children that food is a part of the joy of life rather than an unpleasant chore or a cause for anxiety.

If the following suggestions can be observed, even when there is no immediate danger of an eating disorder, families are more likely to avoid them—and in the process have a good time, too.

At the table

Mealtimes need to be pleasant. Because of frantic schedules these days, having family dinner every night may not be possible, but it's important to make eating food a positive, shared experience at a regular time. Whether it's Sunday brunch or dinner every Thursday, make it a celebration, not an act of endurance. Let each child take turns picking music or deciding the menu. And while the table is certainly a place to learn social skills, the process should be enjoyable for everyone.

Getting everyone into the kitchen

Whether or not you have family dinner every night, you can create positive associations with food by having everyone at one time or another help with the buying and preparing of meals and special treats. Learning to cook helps young children get a sense of mastery over their world—they learn that they *can* take care of themselves in positive ways (as opposed to taking control in a destructive or *self*-destructive way). Cooking together as a family also offers good opportunities for conversation about all kinds of subjects, including ideas about food.

Making exercise fun

Instead of reminding your child when sending her off to play soccer that an athletic scholarship will get her through college, reassure her that any kind of

Bright Idea
Try not to argue at the table when food is being eaten. These negative experiences become associated with eating, and then food itself becomes a problem. In fact, if heavy stuff is discussed *after* eating, people tend to handle it better.

exercise is good for feeling healthy and happy and that healthy bodies and happy people come in all shapes and sizes. The exercise message given to children should be this:

> "Remember: Kids and adults who exercise and stay *active* are healthier and better able to do what they want to do, no matter what they weigh or how they look. Try to find a sport that you like, and do it. It's not about going out for a team, unless you want to. Maybe it's even about walking to school a couple of days a week instead of riding: That's great exercise!"

Rather than focusing on exercise as a competitive sport, exercise should be a fun part of family life. When your kids are involved in sports, let them know that you're proud of *that*—not just winning. Your family should take a little time each day, week, or weekend to get involved in vigorous play that is just plain fun.

This kind of attitude toward exercise can't hurt parents, either, because if the message is going to get across, you'll have to find exercise that *you* enjoy, too. You'll then become good role models in regard to sensible eating, sensible exercise, and self-acceptance.

Eating disorders are really about disordered lives. This type of life can be avoided by putting serious thought into how we can achieve and enjoy a balance in every part of our lives.

Just the Facts

- Thinking carefully about the role food plays in your family life can help prevent eating problems.

- Because food problems tend to express emotional conflicts, do what you can to head off conflicts before they develop into an eating disorder.

- Children who feel good about themselves and know that their parents approve of them don't need to use food as a weapon.

- Food and exercise can be fun and go a long way toward relieving family tensions.

GET THE SCOOP ON...
The body's biochemical balance ▪ Why dieting
doesn't work ▪ Real nutrition facts ▪ What
weight is "ideal"? ▪ Putting it all in motion

In Balance

The best way to prevent disordered eating patterns is to maintain a body that is in balance. However, so much misinformation circulates about what goes into making our bodies work at their best that it is hard to know what is really important.

In the simplest of terms, the body is an energy factory fueled and regulated by chemicals that it both takes in (as food) and produces (as hormones). To survive and thrive, the body depends upon keeping that intake and outgo in balance, and it strenuously resists any efforts to throw it off balance.

Dieting and bingeing throw this chemical factory out of whack, so it's especially important to know how to rebalance and make the best use of what comes in—in the form of food. People in recovery from an eating disorder, especially those who have spent an excessive amount of time and energy obsessively controlling their food intake, need to refocus their attention on learning about and practicing healthy eating.

Chapter 16

The goal is to take in enough food to balance outgo of energy with the maintenance of a body weight that is right for each individual.

Hunger and satiety

Under normal circumstances, people know to eat when they feel hungry and to stop eating when they feel full (or satiated). People who have eating disorders, however, lose the ability to feel these cues. This loss may be partially due to psychological causes, but disordered eating is known to throw the delicate chemical interaction of hunger and fullness off-balance.

Unofficially...
Cholecystokinin (CCK), a hormone known to be deficient in some women who have bulimia, causes laboratory animals to feel full and stop eating.

Hunger and satiety happen in the brain—not in the stomach or gut. To put it simply, the feeling of being hungry or full depends on the level of nutrients and glucose in the blood that stimulate receptors in the stomach lining to secrete hormones that then signal the need for more or less food. Animal studies have shown that simply filling up the stomach with substances that do not produce nutrients or convert to glucose does not stop the animal from eating: Hunger is more than just having a full belly.

As the stomach releases a number of hormones, a complex chemical process alerts the brain to create the sensation of a full stomach. But if no new food is taken in to replenish blood sugar, the chemical adrenaline is released into the body, which ultimately causes the body to release *stored* sugar and to *make* sugar out of protein.

When this process occurs on a regular basis—during self-starvation, for example—it can overburden the body's emergency system and ultimately wear it out. In addition to these basic regulators, other hormones that are also important to the hunger/satiety balance may be rendered ineffective by bingeing and starvation.

This neuroendocrine system—that is, the system that provides the chemicals that create the circuits through which nerves send messages—regulates sexual function, physical growth and development, appetite and digestion, sleep, heart and kidney function, emotions, thinking, and memory. Thus, the purpose of all this chemistry that relies on the intake of food is to keep all body processes running smoothly and to help us stay in balance. The whole process is called metabolism, which means the rate and efficiency at which the body turns food into energy.

The basal metabolic rate, which powers the body's invisible but critical functions, represents nearly three-fourths of all energy expenditure. This is why nutrition—the intake of food—is so important and why inadequate or irregular intake of food seriously interferes with body functions.

Why dieting doesn't work

If the body has a purpose, it is to maintain itself as efficiently as possible so that we can go about the business of life. The body's goal is equilibrium, or balance, so it maintains a set point.

Set point

Set point is the weight range that your body has programmed for you; it is based on your genetic and chemical makeup, and it works very hard to maintain that weight. Set points vary from person to person. For example, two women who are the same height and who have the same frame may think they should weigh the same, but if their set points differ, their bodies will fight to maintain different weights.

Watch Out!
Every bodily function operates according to a communications system of neurotransmitters—chemical substances that transmit nerve impulses between nerve cells. The brain sends electrical signals to every muscle and organ in the body, but these signals will be blocked unless neurotransmitters keep them moving. In essence, neurotransmitters are produced by the digestion of food. More than 300 known neurotransmitters—including endorphins, which contribute to a feeling of emotional well-being; and compounds such as acetylcholine, which regulates the activities of the body's crucial involuntary systems—keep all bodily organs functioning.

The body's metabolism slows down when weight drops below its set point so that any weight loss is slow; likewise, the metabolic process increases when weight rises above the set point. The body tries to fight against the increase in weight by speeding up metabolism and raising its temperature to burn off the unwanted calories.

Apparently, set point also is regulated by body chemistry. The hypothalamus, a center in the brain that regulates the amount of fatty tissue stored by the body, may also determine set point. When this region of the brain detects sufficient amounts of leptin, a chemical that is produced by fat cells and that travels via the blood until it reaches the brain, it tells the body to stop storing fat. When the hypothalamus is cut out of an animal, that animal does not know that it is already "fat enough" and will continue to gain weight—even on a restricted diet!

Off balance

Dieting throws our delicate chemical balance out of whack; consequently, the body works hard to regain and maintain its balance. Human and animal studies reveal that the amount of weight lost during a diet is much less than one might expect, based solely on the reduction of calories. This is because the metabolic rate rises dramatically as caloric intake decreases. In other words, as less food is eaten, the body compensates—in fact, it overcompensates—and becomes more efficient by burning less food. People who are genetically programmed to be heavy maintain increasingly larger fat reserves by eating the same amount, or fewer calories, than people who weigh less naturally.

In the first few weeks of dieting, weight is usually lost. However, it is almost always gained back. After a few weeks of dieting, weight loss usually stops even though food intake is restricted. This is a sign that the body is fighting to retain its natural weight. When dieting continues, the body senses semi-starvation and tries to conserve energy even more dramatically. Dieters may start to sleep more, and body temperature may drop. The urge to binge may be triggered by the body's attempt to restore its metabolic balance.

More chemical matters

Chemical imbalances mean more than the success or failure of diets. Research on the neuroendocrine system has found that these regulatory mechanisms, which are linked to mood and depression, are seriously disturbed in many people who have eating disorders. Mood disorders run in families, so further study is being done to explore the links between depression and eating disorders.

Similar chemical imbalances have been found in people who have eating disorders and those who have other conditions, such as addiction and obsessive/compulsive disorder. Although no conclusive evidence exists, it is just as likely that inadequate chemical intake due to disordered eating patterns causes emotional problems.

While many eating disorder specialists have great hopes for the effectiveness of biochemical treatments, research is still in the beginning stages. Other than using antidepressants, most specialists still consider it better to normalize eating patterns without introducing external chemicals.

But the results of biochemical research could lead to enhanced treatments for eating disorders. Beyond that, these findings demonstrate that eating disorders truly are disorders, not just willful misbehavior.

Unofficially...
A recent study suggests that a drop in levels of the neurotransmitter serotonin and its precursor, tryptophan, may trigger symptoms of bulimia in vulnerable individuals. It works like this: Healthy adult women who diet may experience a reduction of serotonin, which then may trigger the cycle of bingeing and purging.
—*Archives of General Psychiatry*, 1999

Still, even when chemical therapy helps relieve the symptoms of eating disorders, most professionals—as well as the patients who are in recovery—feel that psychological, educational, and emotional support are just as important for a full recovery from eating disorders.

Moneysaver
A lot of the best nutrition advice is available free from the federal government. See Appendix B for contact information.

The basics of a healthful diet

While each body has its own needs and its own chemistry, anyone can make use of certain fundamentals. Eating probably shouldn't be made into a "project"—indeed, eating-disorder counselors are wary of encouraging their clients to devote too much energy even to healthy eating—but good nutrition is something that needs to be learned to become habit. Although individual patients should get advice from their doctors about what they should eat to maintain their health, a few good general guidelines exist.

Positive eating strategies

Again, anyone who is in recovery from an eating disorder should get dietary guidelines from the therapists and nutritionists overseeing their recovery; these professionals are best equipped to help patients devise food plans and establish and maintain weight goals.

This chapter contains several strategies to help meet these goals, not only for recovering people but also for the families and friends who are involved in their lives. The no-dieting view of healthy eating might also be of value because of its emphasis on maintaining a flexible balance.

When allowed to follow a natural course and establish its own balance, the body sends cues for the calories it needs to cover the amount of energy expended in exercise and what is needed for maintenance and repair. In other words, if we become attuned to the natural balance of our body's needs, we'll know *when* it's time to eat. This attunement helps us maintain a weight within our body's set point and allows us to pay attention to other issues. This may be hard to believe for anyone who has thoroughly bought into today's dieting culture, but it *is* how the body really works.

The right kind of attention

Ideally, we shouldn't have to think too much about what we are doing to give ourselves sufficient calories and nutrients. We should simply be able do what comes naturally and eat what's best for us. However this can be something of a challenge in our food- and diet-obsessed culture, especially for people who are recovering from an eating disorder and for whom it is essential to maintain a healthy balance of calories and nutrients.

Natural regulation

An important part of the treatment of eating disorders is to eat at consistently regular intervals. When this pattern is followed on a day-to-day basis, the body regulates itself. Hunger is experienced in a regular pattern, and the body can maintain its own balance.

Building a diet on good nutrition

You do have to plan for a well-balanced nutritional program, especially if you are beginning a new way of life. But food planning can be fun and satisfying when the goal is to make your body feel good rather than miserable or deprived. Where the objective of food planning once was to keep intake so low that the body starved itself, now the goal is to make it glow with energy and well-being.

The Food Guide Pyramid

Although the federal government has developed food plans to meet nutritional requirements, continuing research leads them to update recommendations periodically. The government's current guidelines, which require manufacturers to print information about nutrition on the labels of most packaged foods, are designed to help you select food for an eating plan that will meet the guidelines recommended in the Food Guide Pyramid.

This Pyramid is meant for all healthy people from age 2 on up. It offers practical advice to enjoy the diverse array of foods available in today's marketplace. In its five food groups, the Pyramid offers many kinds of foods that promote health. Chosen carefully, all foods can be part of a healthy eating style. Follow the Pyramid's advice: You'll get all the nutrients and energy you need, without too many calories or too much fat, cholesterol, or sugars. Enjoy your favorite foods and favorite places to eat. After all, no foods or meals are "good" or "bad." The foods you choose for the whole day or even several

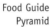

Food Guide
Pyramid

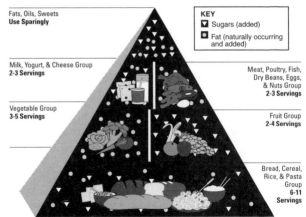

Fats, Oils, Sweets
Use Sparingly

KEY
☑ Sugars (added)
▣ Fat (naturally occurring and added)

Milk, Yogurt, & Cheese Group
2-3 Servings

Meat, Poultry, Fish, Dry Beans, Eggs, & Nuts Group
2-3 Servings

Vegetable Group
3-5 Servings

Fruit Group
2-4 Servings

Bread, Cereal, Rice, & Pasta Group
6-11 Servings

SOURCE: U.S. Department of Agriculture/U.S. Department of Health and Human Services

days are what count, so don't worry if a particular meal isn't as balanced as it could be. And remember that it's okay to enjoy just a bit from the tip of the Pyramid, too!

Balancing food groups

Of course, no single food can supply all nutrients in the amounts you need. For example, oranges provide vitamin C but no vitamin B; cheese provides vitamin B but no vitamin C. To make sure you get all the nutrients and other substances needed for good health, try to eat at least the lowest number of servings from each of the five major food groups each day. Choosing a variety of foods improves the diet because foods within the same group offer different combinations of nutrients as well as other beneficial substances. For example, some vegetables and fruits within the same group might be good sources of vitamin C or vitamin A, while others might offer good supplies of calcium or iron. Choosing a variety of foods from each group also helps to make meals more interesting and satiating from day to day.

Here's a quick but important caveat about food fads: Almost every issue of every popular magazine has an article about some new food fact. But more often than not, these "facts" are just stories about fads that have no basis in fact—or, they're "news" that has emerged from studies that are less than conclusive. If you follow the press for information about any new food fad or breakthrough for more than a few months, you'll learn that you should "never" eat fat, or eat only "good" fat, or eat only "some" fat, or—oh well, never mind.

Keep it simple, and keep it basic: Eat some fat, some protein, some carbohydrates, and five fruits and vegetables a day. All that's really needed is to follow some fairly simple guidelines.

Unofficially...
There is so much information about food, and so much of it is conflicting or erroneous, that the best source for nutrition advice may be a professional nutritionist. He not only has accurate facts, but he also can gear advice to your special needs.

Nondieting guidelines

These guidelines from eating-disorder professionals can be of great use not only to the people we know who are in recovery, but also to all of us who have absorbed cultural diet messages since childhood:

- Let hunger be your guide to *when* you eat and satiety your cue to stop.

- Enjoy a variety of foods from all food groups.

- Select foods you'll enjoy eating within the general framework of three meals a day, plus some snacks.

- There's nothing wrong with eating to celebrate, eating for comfort, or eating for fun.

- Don't feel compelled to clean your plate—or to have seconds—but, on the other hand, don't be afraid to have more when something is really delicious.

- Pay attention to what you eat, and plan meals for nutritional value—but remember that what you may miss today will balance out over the longer term.

- Be flexible about when, where, and under what circumstances you eat.

If there are any foods to avoid, it's an overabundance of both high-sugar and sugar-*free* diet products. These add no nutrition to the body and may have the effect of throwing off the natural appetite. Likewise, caffeine and alcohol are best taken in moderation.

Are all calories alike?

Generally speaking, all calories—whether from carbohydrates, proteins, fats, or alcohol—supply the same amount of energy. However, each source

---

Understanding Calories

Calories are units of energy contained in the foods we eat. The components in foods that provide calories are carbohydrates, proteins, fats, and alcohol. Each of these components provides the following number of calories *per gram:*

Carbohydrate	4 calories per gram
Protein	4 calories per gram
Fat	9 calories per gram
Alcohol	7 calories per gram

1 gram weighs about as much as a safety pin

---

provides unique contributions to bodily function and health.

Carbohydrates

Foods high in carbohydrates (including breads and starches) are mostly used for energy. The fiber in many high-carbohydrate foods also helps regulate bowel function and protects against heart disease and certain types of cancer. Carbohydrates should make up about 60 percent of your total daily calories.

Protein

Protein in foods (including meat, dairy, and soybean products) are used for energy, but the body also uses protein to make and maintain body tissue, such as muscles and organs. In addition, protein is a key component of enzymes and hormones, among other body fluids. When the body takes in enough calories from other sources, it uses protein for these essential purposes rather than for fuel. Only about 15 percent of your daily calories should come from protein.

Fat

Fat (which includes butter and animal fats) provides the most concentrated source of energy. Even a little fat can provide a lot of calories. Fat comes in two forms: saturated and unsaturated. Saturated fats, which usually are from animal sources, can absorb nothing, so they are more likely to clog the arteries than unsaturated fats, which usually are from plants. No more than 30 percent of your daily calories should come from fat (unsaturated is probably a healthier choice than saturated).

Alcohol

Alcohol also provides a concentrated source of calories. In excess, it can alter judgment, lead to dependency, and cause other serious health problems. Alcohol can increase appetite and decrease will power, which contributes to overeating—even more unwanted calories!

To sum it up, health professionals recommend a balance of these energy sources: Up to 60 percent of your daily calories should come from carbohydrates, about 15 percent from protein, and no more than 30 percent from fat. Alcohol is not recommended as a source of calories.

How many calories do you need?

Caloric needs vary considerably from one individual to another. A small, elderly, and sedentary woman requires fewer calories than a large, young, physically active man does. A growing teenage girl who is active in sports, a pregnant woman, or a woman athlete needs more calories than a young woman who has an office job. In other words, the number of calories you need depends on your age, height, weight, sex, and activity level. Although all these factors determine energy requirements, it is possible to estimate your approximate calorie needs by multiplying your weight in pounds by 12. Remember that this is only a rough estimate, and many people who are in recovery from anorexia still need to gain weight to maintain good health.

It's also important to know that calories can take a wide variety of forms and accommodate a wide range in taste. All kinds of interesting choices can be made with the same number of calories: a 350-calorie breakfast, for instance, might consist of yogurt, mixed fruit, and whole-wheat toast—or it could be pancakes and ham!

Likewise, a 500-calorie dinner might be a steak and a potato, or rice and beans. In sum, anyone can make eating both healthy and enjoyable.

Why it's important to plan meals

Everyone needs to plan meals, not only people who are trying to regain nutritional balance after an eating disorder. Many people go to professional nutritionists for dietary advice as part of their overall healthcare program, in part because food and the food industry have become so complex and inscrutable these days. It is hard to know sometimes what is actually in some foods!

An eating plan is not a diet. Anyone who wants to stay healthy needs practice in developing food and eating patterns that provide nutritional needs as well as enjoyment. Some people need special guidance in doing this: For example, people who are in recovery from anorexia are advised to make a point of *not* being careful about some things (such as French fries) but must be careful, on other hand, about not drinking diet drinks. Whether or not you have an eating disorder, you can find professional help for these eating plans in the resources listed at the back of this book (see Appendix B, "Resource Guide"). Parents who are trying to get their children's eating patterns back on track (whether following treatment for an eating disorder or as a way to prevent them) will find this information helpful, too.

Determining an ideal weight

Even doctors who specialize in weight and eating have a hard time determining the ideal weight for individuals in their care. This difficulty does not stem from lack of knowledge, but from an understanding that weights vary widely among individuals.

Today the consensus among professionals who specialize in eating disorders is that assigning weights to people according to insurance company charts (which was done for years!) makes as much sense as assigning heights according to a chart. It is now generally acknowledged that insurance chart rates are based on averages and that nobody in particular seems to fit them. Consequently, doctors take into account height, bone structure, and healthy levels of body fat to evaluate the right weight for a person. Or, after taking a patient's medical history, a doctor may be able to establish her set point, or natural range within which her weight might be expected to fluctuate. To establish a set point for yourself, the best advice is to eat normally and exercise moderately. After a period of maintaining this natural pattern of eating and exercising (it may take up to a month for people whose eating has been disordered), your body will settle into a weight range that is healthy for you.

Body Mass Index (BMI)

Another weight guideline that has gained popularity and which doctors feel is more valuable (and safer) than weight-and-measurement charts is the Body Mass Index (BMI).

The BMI is a ratio of weight to height that, when calculated, produces a key number that indicates if a person is within a healthy weight range. The BMI is found by multiplying your weight in pounds by 703, mulitiplying your height in inches by itself, then dividing the first number by the second. BMIs from nineteen to twenty-five indicate a healthy weight. However, this form of measurement can't be viewed as absolute (any more than weight-and-measurement charts can) because it doesn't take into account muscularity or bone density. For example, a large-boned or muscular person may have a BMI that reads "too high" but that is actually healthy; someone who has smaller bones and less muscle weight may have a BMI rate that looks healthy but is actually too low.

Nevertheless, the BMI is viewed by health professionals as a valuable measure of body composition because it correlates highly with body fat in *most* people.

An additional measurement is waist circumference, which can provide additional guidelines either for those who are extremely fit and muscular or for those whose light frame and overabundance of fat may fool the BMI. The waist circumference is measured around a person's natural waist (just above the navel). A waist circumference of 35 inches or more for women, or 40 inches or more for men is considered to indicate overweight, no matter what the BMI.

Physicians, however, are more concerned with other indicators of health, such as measurements of blood pressure and cholesterol, and with habits

Watch Out! The fact that a well-exercised body is more muscular is a catch-22 for compulsive dieters and exercisers. The more they exercise, the heavier their bodies may become because muscle weighs more than fat. This imbalance drives some dieters to extremes. Likewise, poor nutrition can eat away at bones, so any weight loss that occurs results in fragile bones.

How to Determine Body Mass Index

Use these steps to calculate your BMI. A calculator will help.

1. Measure height and weight

2. Multiply weight in pounds by 703

3. Divide by height in inches

4. Divide again by height in inches.

For example: a 5-foot person who weights 100 pounds calculates BMI this way: $100 \times 703 = 70300$, divided by $60 = 1171.6$, divided by $60 = 19.5$. The BMI is 19.5

Weight specialists consider BMI values less than 19 underweight; BMI values from 19 to 25 normal; BMI from 26 to 30 as overweight; and BMI from 31 to 39 as very overweight. BMI of 40 and above is considered extremely overweight.

For help in calculating and interpreting your BMI, visit the Web site of Shape Up, America! at www.shapeup.org.

such as smoking and exercise, than they are with ideal weights. Increasingly, it's becoming clear that Americans' ideas about beautiful bodies are market-driven instead of based on sound health.

Some specialists on eating disorders consider the ideal weight one that can be maintained comfortably without diet restrictions. This should appeal to a lot of people who are tired of worrying about their weight!

Of course, within that definition, it *is* possible to be truly too fat or too thin—that is, so heavy or so underweight naturally that body functions are impaired. A physician is the best judge of this. Doctors who have not been negatively influenced by the media's preference for and idealization of slim bodies probably won't be concerned about under or overweight as long as cholesterol, blood pressure, and blood chemistry are within normal ranges. But when any of these indicators enters the danger zone, weight definitely becomes an issue, especially when other risk factors such as smoking or a family history of eating disorders and related problems is present.

The exercise factor

The best attitude toward food is one that incorporates healthful eating into an active lifestyle. The whole point of eating is to live in a body that allows you to do interesting and often energetic things and to feel at ease about doing them. It's also true that the human body is designed to work better if it's well exercised.

Exercise keeps weight in balance by expending energy, and it reduces fat storage by altering the leptin mechanism. Therefore, finding a way to work 30 minutes of fairly vigorous exercise—enough to make you breathe a little hard or sweat a bit—into most days of the week is what's needed to maintain your chemical balance and a weight that's right for you.

Exercise, of course, can also be deeply satisfying and enjoyable in itself. It even has been documented that exercise can stir up a remarkably heady chemical cocktail. Runners, in particular, report that they feel refreshed, invigorated, and even "high" after some runs, apparently because of the release of certain brain chemicals that induce a feeling of well-being.

Certain kinds of exercise reduce stress and enhance mood as well. Rhythmic exercises, such as rowing, increase brain activity that produces a calm state similar to meditation. Almost any level of exercise can lead to the release of serotonin, the brain chemical that contributes to feelings of relaxation and satisfaction. Vigorous exercise causes the brain to release endorphins, which ease pain and provide an even stronger sense of well-being. Apart from the chemical benefits, exercise provides a distraction from stress, stimulates creativity, and inspires something as simple and basic as having fun. What a concept!

Just the Facts

- The body's chemical composition is complex and subtle, but eating a variety of foods can help keep it in balance.

- A basic knowledge of nutrition gives you lots of freedom to eat healthfully—and enjoy it, too.

- Give yourself a general idea of the calories you need for basic maintenance, and then eat what you enjoy.

- Eating the right amount of the right foods—for you—and getting the right amount of exercise that is enjoyable—for you—will help keep your health in balance.

GET THE SCOOP ON...
The outlook for recovery ▪ Facts to remember ▪
Keys to success ▪ What recovery feels like

Chapter 17

Looking Ahead

There's good news about eating disorders, as the information gathered in this book indicates. These disorders are treatable, and they are preventable. Although the causes—as well as the psychological and physiological processes that govern the disorders—are intricate and complex, there are fairly simple steps to take toward recovery from them.

Improving the outlook

No matter what the approach to recovery, similar steps are involved, beginning with an awareness of the problem and the willingness to accept treatment.

Once in treatment, a patient with an eating disorder must first be helped to stabilize eating patterns. When a fairly healthy balance is restored, it may be time to explore in-depth causes and then establish new patterns of eating and exercise.

Put this way, recovery sounds simple. In a sense, it *is* a simple step-by-step process—but "simple" does not necessarily mean "easy."

Facts to remember

Successful recovery starts with facing facts and moving beyond them. Here are some important ones to remember:

- Anorexia, bulimia, binge eating, and other eating disorders are the products of a combination of psychological, physiological, familial, and social factors.

- Eating disorders are physical compulsions driven by mental obsessions that serve as powerful tools in an individual's struggle for self-expression.

- The influence of mass media on how we perceive images of the body has a demonstrable effect on we feel about our own bodies. Ideal body types promoted by the media are far slimmer and leaner than normal and may not even be healthy for most people.

- Distorted body perceptions begin very early in life and affect children's feelings about themselves. A direct connection exists between body image distortion and the severity of an eating disorder.

- People in modern Western cultures automatically face confusion about food and eating habits due to the proliferation of commercial versus medical messages about diet. In this context, a serious eating disorder may be difficult to spot.

- If an eating disorder is suspected, it probably exists.

- Understanding the causes of eating disorders is critical, but often the causes are subtle, under the surface, and not immediately clear to either the sufferer or her family and friends.

- Eating disorders have more to do with intense emotions turned inward, due to deep feelings of inadequacy, than they do about food.

- The most common trigger for an eating disorder is a weight-loss diet.

- Eating disorders *can* be treated successfully, and the earlier the better. Successful treatment depends on tailoring tested approaches to individual needs.

- Effective treatment changes a patient's eating patterns, psychological responses, and body perceptions. The process may be brief or lengthy, with a single professional or a team, but it can achieve success through a careful, step-by-step course. Almost any school of therapy can treat eating disorders.

- Finding cost-effective therapy is possible, and free information and support networks are easy to tap into.

- The pain of living with or being close to someone who has an eating disorder is real, but there are steps to take to ameliorate the physical and emotional effects of living with someone who has an eating disorder.

- Family and friends can be supportive without giving in or pandering to an eating disorder.

- If you live with someone who has an eating disorder, getting help for yourself can help the sufferer—and make your own life more worthwhile, too.

- Families and friends have a variety of choices for support and treatment; whether families are asked to come into the therapeutic process or not, they may benefit from getting help themselves.

■ Coming to accept the fact that physical appearance is not the key to personal worth—and that our bodies are naturally calibrated to be at a certain weight—are good ways to prevent and stop vicious cycles of dieting. The harder the effort to go below the body's set point range, the harder the body will fight to retain its natural weight.

■ "Normal" relationships with food are ones in which both intake and outgo are balanced in moderation.

■ Eating the right amount of the right foods—*for you*—and getting the right amount of the most enjoyable kinds of exercise—*for you*—keep body and mind in balance.

Keys to recovery

As we learn more about eating disorders and experiment with different types of therapy, the outlook for recovery improves. On an individual basis, however, we can isolate a variety of factors that influence a positive outcome. For example, specialists in treating eating disorders note these points:

1. The biggest positive influence in recovery is a strong desire to give up the disorder, no matter what the perceived cost, fears of gaining weight, control surrendered, or anxiety-producing foods eaten.

2. A responsive support system ranks next. This means that if a person who has an eating disorder is living at home, his family must be willing to enter treatment themselves to examine

A woman with a nine-year history of chronic anorexia and who had been hospitalized many times found a job that she loved and eventually let go of her eating disorder. The desire to work and feel good about herself helped to pull her away from the illness.

behaviors and attitudes that might have contributed to the person's illness. Or it means having friends who are willing to listen and also to demonstrate anxiety-free eating. In either case, it's important to lean on people who won't force or pressure those with an eating disorder to change.

3. It is important for people who are in recovery to have other areas of their lives that work well—and activities that they're proud of and to which they are committed.

4. Having goals outside the illness is very important. Some people define themselves by their disorder, and eventually their lives become centered on being sick. For others, hopes and dreams to marry and have children, for example, or to become a doctor help to pull them away from the illness as they move toward their goals.

What it means to recover

With so much research underway, and with the wide general awareness and acceptance of eating disorders as serious but treatable conditions, prospects for recovery are generally very good and will only get better as we learn more about both the underlying causes of eating disorders and their treatment.

> " The eating disorder has changed the way I look at the world. Going though the hard work of recovery has caused me to grow. I'm finally really moving on.
> —A young woman who now describes herself as intelligent, strong, resilient, beautiful, and creative "

Already a great deal has been learned about recovery from the people who have gone through it themselves. Even people who are in the throes of a devastating disorder have reason for hope.

From an even more positive viewpoint, some people on the other side of eating disorders summarize their painful experiences as a turning point, the beginning of a journey to a fuller and more rewarding life. Like many people who have experienced life-threatening dangers, they come to value life highly. That's another piece of good news related to eating disorders: After recovery, people find that their lives are even richer.

From the beginning

People begin recovery by talking about what it was like to be in the grip of an eating disorder. They talk about the agony of anorexia and bulimia and relate what it's like to think constantly about food and to step on the scale many times a day. They describe the guilt of eating, the horror of not being able to stop, the pressure to exercise, and the triumph of not eating. They tell about how lonely it can feel, the hundred little distortions that help hide the eating disorder, and getting to the point where death seems like a better option than another day of misery: "I wasn't living," they say. "I was in hell."

In despair, some people reach out to eating disorder support groups. From there, they find treatment. It's scary, the survivors say. It *is* hard to imagine a life without counting calories and purging; it's hard to let go of "the one thing that keeps you going, that organizes the day, that provides purpose."

As recovery begins, the survivors describe how hard it is to binge and finally not purge, or to feel the terror of gaining weight and feeling clothes grow tighter. Then they describe the fear of experiencing feelings that have been numb for so long. They say that recovery brings guilt, fear, and sadness, not to mention the sheer frustration of getting better. However, the consensus is that *it's all worth it*.

Inevitably, there is talk about how hard therapy can be, that recovery is "something other people do," and that the process might go on forever because they can't imagine letting go of the control they once had over their lives. It is also difficult to shake the belief that by controlling the food that went into their bodies, they were able to make their own lives (and those of others) much more manageable. Unlearning this is tough. Once, seeing the pain they caused other people only made them try all the more to control themselves. Now, the difficulty is letting go of control.

The value of support

It wouldn't be possible to break out of any of these vicious circles without *support*, people in recovery say. They admit that it takes a long time to learn to enjoy oneself again and to relax from so much inner rigidity. But they tell others who are considering recovery that once they've gotten to the other side, they won't believe that they've spent so much time with an eating disorder. In recovery, they find life wonderful and exciting again, if a little scary in the beginning. They see, perhaps for the first time, just how bleak their lives had been. Whether they are feeling full of life and energy or simply enjoying the pleasures of thicker, shinier hair, people in recovery say that it is worth every ounce of effort. Finally learning to love their bodies is perhaps the most positive aspect of getting better: They are happy to

> **❝**
> After a while, you have to stop defining yourself as someone who has an eating disorder. You have to decide at some point that that was you *then*, but this is you *now*.
> —A young woman in recovery
> **❞**

have the energy and desire to make full use of them once again.

Whatever their condition or circumstances, people don't have to go through recovery by themselves. Support and information is plentiful, as the Appendix B, "Resource Guide," shows.

Just the Facts

- Rates of recovery vary, depending on the nature of the eating disorder and the background of the sufferer.

- Research is increasing the odds in favor of recovery.

- People who are determined to get better and who have positive goals are most likely to succeed.

- The results of recovery are definitely worth the effort.

Glossary

12-step method System of recovery based on techniques proven successful in Alcoholics Anonymous, developed from the idea of being "powerless" over the compulsions and seeking help to move away from them.

addiction Irresistible physiological and/or psychological need for a habit-forming substance or behavior.

amenorrhea Absence of menstrual periods.

anorexia nervosa An eating disorder characterized by: refusal to maintain normal body weight; intense fear of gaining weight, body image distortion, and amenorrhea. Two types of anorexia exist: restricting, which involves self-starvation without bingeing or purging; and binge eating/purging, where binges or purges are added to dieting.

athletica nervosa Compulsive overexercising.

BED (Binge Eating Disorder) An eating disorder characterized by recurrent episodes of bingeing—that is, eating large quantities of food more rapidly than normal until uncomfortably full and when not hungry. Bingeing episodes cause distress and are *not* followed by any type of purge.

behavioral psychology A form of psychotherapy that uses basic learning techniques to modify maladaptive behavior patterns by substituting new responses to given stimuli for undesirable ones.

binge eating The consumption of an unusually large quantity of food within a brief period of time. It can occur within the context of any eating disorder, as well as in nonpathological situations.

Body Mass Index (BMI) A ratio of weight to height that, when calculated, may more accurately determing whether a person is obese than does that person's weight on a scale.

bulimarexia A combination of bulimia and anorexia, an eating disorder in which one alternates between abnormal craving for and aversion to food. It is characterized by episodes of excessive food intake followed by periods of fasting and self-induced vomiting or diarrhea.

bulimia nervosa Insatiable appetite eating disorder characterized by recurrent episodes of bingeing followed by compensatory behavior to prevent weight gain. Bingeing techniques can include vomiting; use of laxatives, diuretics, or enemas; and/or excessive exercise.

calorie Quantity of heat required to raise the temperature of 1 gram of water by 1°C from a standard initial temperature; a unit of energy contained in food, as measured by actually burning food in a calorimeter.

chronic dieter A person whose disordered eating involves keeping careful track of foods selected from a limited list, focusing on those that will help lose weight and avoiding those that might cause weight gain. Chronic dieters conscientiously exercise at least once or twice a day and weigh daily; while they probably don't fit a strict eating-disorder diagnosis, their focus on food intake is maladaptive.

CBT (Cognitive Behavioral Therapy) A form of psychological therapy that focuses on an individual's ability to learn new behaviors.

compulsion An irresistible impulse to commit an irrational act. Compulsive overeating, for example, implies people who use food to manage stress and difficult emotions, and who overeat even though their worries about their weight make overeating irrational.

denial In psychology, an unconscious defense mechanism characterized by refusal to acknowledge painful realities, thoughts, or feelings; refusing to believe what is actual.

dieting Avoiding eating for long periods of time (in other words, starving, which may lead to bingeing); avoiding eating certain types of food (craving, which may lead to bingeing), and restricting the total amount of food eaten (starving, which may lead to bingeing).

diuretic A substance or drug that tends to increase the discharge of urine used by people with eating disorders in the mistaken belief that it prevents weight gain. As with laxatives, individuals may feel that they've lost weight due to the resulting dehydration. Abuse of diuretics can easily result in depletion of important electrolytes, sodium, and potassium.

dehydration Lack of fluid in the body, resulting in feelings of dizziness and weakness accompanied by low blood pressure and fast heart rate. When prolonged, it can cause serious physical damage.

eating disorders Any of several psychological disorders relating to the consumption of food, such as

anorexia nervosa and bulimia. They are characterized by an abnormal fear of obesity, distorted body
image, and subsequent abnormal eating patterns.

ED-NOS   Eating Disorder, Not Otherwise Specified. Because eating disorders come in so many variations, another new definition has been devised to
cover those disordered food-related patterns that do
not fit standard diagnoses. Symptoms nearly fitting
criteria for other disorders qualify as ED-NOS, as
does the pattern of chewing and spitting out large
amounts of food without swallowing.

electrolytes   Electrical conductors in which current
is carried by ions (as in the body) rather than by free
electrons (as in a metal). Physiological electrolytes,
whose function is to communicate nerve messages
throughout all the systems of the body, include
water solutions of salts and other minerals, such as
sodium and potassium. When sodium is low due to
dehydration or starvation, the result is lethargy and
weakness, which progresses to seizures. Low potassium levels lead to cardiac conduction defects,
arrhythmias, skeletal and smooth muscle weakness,
and decreased gastrointestinal motility

emetic   A substance that causes vomiting.

endorphins   Any of a group of neurotransmitters
that affect mood, perception of pain, memory retention, and learning. Their appropriate chemical
makeup requires the ingestion of a balanced diet.

family therapy   A form of psychotherapy in which
the interrelationships of family members are exam-
ined in group sessions to identify and alleviate the
problems of one or more members of the family.

Food Guide Pyramid   The combination of dietary
allowances recommended by nutritionists and supported by U.S. government research.

hormones Chemical messengers released in small but essential amounts by the body's endocrine glands. Each hormone has a specific function, and each is carried by the bloodstream to the tissues or organs it regulates. Inadequate nutrition creates inadequate production of hormones, thus affecting each organ in the body.

laxative A food or drug that causes looseness or evacuation of the bowels; used by people who have eating disorders to purge food from the body in an attempt to avoid caloric intake. This attempt is ineffective because the drugs primarily affect the large intestine, whereas most nutrients are absorbed in the small intestine.

medical nutrition therapy The use of specific nutrition services to treat an illness, injury, or condition. It includes diet therapy, counseling, or use of specialized nutrition supplements.

metabolism The interaction of physical and chemical processes occurring within a living cell or organism that are necessary for the maintenance of life. In human metabolism, substances derived from food are broken down into basic substances to yield energy both for activity and for vital organic processes.

neuroendocrine system Of, relating to, or involving the interaction between the nervous system and the hormones of the endocrine glands.

neurotransmitters Chemicals that transmit information across the junction (synapse) that separates one nerve cell (neuron) from another nerve cell or muscle. More than 300 known neurotransmitters exist in the human body, and each is vital to all bodily functions.

obsession Compulsive preoccupation with a fixed idea or an unwanted feeling or emotion, often accompanied by symptoms of anxiety; also, an intense, often unreasonable idea or emotion.

obsessive-compulsive behaviors   A pattern of pre-occupation with perfectionism and mental and interpersonal control at the expense of flexibility, openness, and efficiency. Eating disorders involve obsessive-compulsive behaviors. That is, sufferers experience a compulsion—an irresistible inner force—to commit an irrational act and are fueled by an obsession—a persistent, unshakable idea that is rooted in an unhealthy mental or emotional state.

Overeaters Anonymous   A mutual self-help, support, and recovery program for people who have eating disorders, based on the 12-step system developed by Alcoholics Anonymous. Their program features regularly scheduled meetings without professional leadership, but with interaction with other sufferers.

psychonutritional therapy   An approach to the treatment of eating disorders in which psychotherapy and medical-nutrition therapy carry through the entire recovery process.

psychopharmacology   The branch of pharmacology that deals with the study of the actions and effects of psychoactive drugs and their application. Eating disorder therapy may involve the use of psychoactive drugs, especially when other conditions such as depression are present.

purge   To cause emptying of the bowels or other segments of the digestive tract through the use of laxatives, emetics, or self-induced vomiting.

relapse   Regarding eating disorders, a regression into the symptoms and behavior of the disorder.

satiety   The condition or sense of being full or gratified. In physiological terms, biochemical signals stimulate the brain in ways that, under normal circumstances, result in the cessation of eating.

set point   The weight range within which a body is programmed by genetics and other factors to weigh.

vomiting   Regurgitation of partially digested foods. In bulimia, this is used as a method of weight control and is caused either by self-stimulation or emetics employed as soon as possible after eating to minimize the absorption of food.

Resource Guide

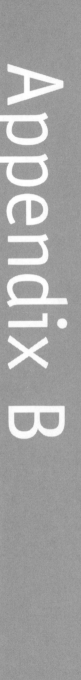

T he number of organizations and Web sites devoted to eating disorders grows steadily. Although some, such as those listed here, are useful and reliable resources, others take advantage of the vulnerability of people who have eating disorders instead of offering assistance; these should be avoided completely. Be especially wary of any group that sells products or services.

Organizations and associations

Each organization listed here provides information, references, and support at no cost.

> The American Anorexia/Bulimia Association, Inc. (AABA)
> 165 W. 46th St.
> New York, NY 10035
> 212-575-6200
> www.aabainc.org

> American Dietetic Association (ADA)
> 16 W. Jackson Blvd.
> Chicago, IL 60606
> 1-800-877-1600
> www.eatright.org

Anorexia Nervosa and Related Eating
Disorders (ANRED)
Box 5102
Eugene, OR 97405
541-344-1144
www.anred.com

Association for Advancement of
Behavior Therapy
305 Seventh Ave.
New York, NY 10001
1-800-685-2228

Bulimia Anorexia Self Help, Inc. (BASH)
6125 Clayton Ave., Suite 215
St. Louis, MO 63139
314-567-4080

Center for the Study of Anorexia and Bulimia
1 W. 91st St.
New York, NY 10024
212-595-3449

Eating Disorders Awareness and Prevention
(EDAP)
603 Stewart St.
Seattle, WA 98101
206-382-3587
www.edap.org

Foundation for Education about Eating
Disorders (FEED)
P.O. Box 16375
Baltimore, MD 21210
410-467-0603

Massachusetts Eating Disorders Association
(MEDA)
92 Pearl St.
Newton, MA 02458
617-558-1881

National Association of Anorexia Nervosa
and Associated Disorders (ANAD)
P.O. Box 7
Highland Park, IL 60035
847-831-3438
www.anad.org

The National Eating Disorders Organization
(NEDO)
6655 South Yale Ave.
Tulsa, OK 74136
918-481-4044
www.nedo.org

National Mental Health Association
1021 Prince St.
Alexandria, VA 22314-2971
1-800-969-6642
www.nmha.org

Overeaters Anonymous
P.O. Box 92870
Los Angeles, CA 90009
310-618-8835
www.overeatersanonymous.org

U.S. Department of Health and
Human Services
P.O. Box 1133
Washington, DC 20013-1133
1-800-336-4797

National Health Information Center
www.nhic-nt.health.org

Web sites

In addition to the Web sites of reputable organizations, such as those listed previously, there are sites
that exist only in cyberspace and that are not supported by any established group. Some people start

Web sites to share their experiences and to network with others. Some are maintained by people seeking to sell their books and services—and even to offer "treatment" via cyberspace. Others that pop up during the course of a Net search and that use "eating disorder" as keywords are actually diet centers! Good judgment is required, as elsewhere on the Internet, before getting too involved with any individual or activity at a Web site.

The following Web sites, however, are particularly valuable, both for their content and for the links they provide to other usually reliable Net resources:

> http://www.something-fishy.org
>
> http://www.mirror-mirror.org
>
> http://www.about-face.org

Books

Hundreds of books on the market are related to eating disorders. Just as with Web sites, these need to be approached with caution. Be skeptical of any that promise cures—especially those that recommend special dietary approaches of any kind. The titles listed here cover specific aspects of eating disorders and are recommended by professionals in the field.

Fairburn, Christopher. *Overcoming Binge Eating.* Guilford Press, 1995.

Friedman, Sandra. *When Girls Feel Fat: Helping Girls through Adolescence.* HarperCollins, 1998.

Hollis, Judi. *Fat Is a Family Affair.* Hazelden, 1996.

Newman, Leslea (Ed.). *Eating Our Hearts Out: Personal Accounts of Women's Relationship to Food.* Crossing Press, 1993.

Sigele, Michelle, Judith Brisman, and Margot
   Weinshel. *Surviving an Eating Disorder:
   Strategies for Family & Friends.* HarperCollins,
   1997.

Treasure, Janet. *Anorexia Nervosa: A Survival Guide
   for Families, Friends, & Sufferers.* Psychology
   Press, 1997.

Zerbe, Kathryn J. *The Body Betrayed: A Deeper
   Understanding of Women, Eating Disorders, and
   Treatment.* Gurze Books, 1995.

For teens and children

Bode, Janet. *Food Fight: A Guide to Eating Disorders
   for Preteens and Their Parents.* Aladdin, 1998.

Davis, Brangien. *What's Real, What's Ideal:
   Overcoming a Negative Body Image.* Rosen
   Publishing Group, 1998.

Levenkron, Steven. *The Best Little Girl in the World.*
   Warner Books, 1981.

Tattersall, Clare. *Understanding Food and Your
   Family.* Rosen Publishing Group, 1999.

An outstanding source for books and other publications for young people, lay people, and professionals is this publisher, which produces material
exclusively related to eating disorders:

Gurze Books
P.O. Box 2238
Carlsbad, CA 92018
1-800-756-7533
www.gurze.com

Send for a free catalog that also lists its news-
letter, information groups, and treatment centers.

A

The *Unofficial Guide*™ Reader Questionnaire

If you would like to express your opinion about starting a business online or this guide, please complete this questionnaire and mail it to:

The *Unofficial Guide*™ Reader Questionnaire
IDG Lifestyle Group
1633 Broadway, floor 7
New York, NY 10019-6785

Gender: ___ M   ___ F

Age: ___ Under 30   ___ 31–40   ___ 41–50
___ Over 50

Education: ___ High school   ___ College
___ Graduate/Professional

What is your occupation?
_____

How did you hear about this guide?
___ Friend or relative
___ Newspaper, magazine, or Internet
___ Radio or TV
___ Recommended at bookstore
___ Recommended by librarian
___ Picked it up on my own
___ Familiar with the *Unofficial Guide*™ series

Did you go to the bookstore specifically for a book on eating disorders?   Yes ___   No ___

Have you used any other *Unofficial Guides*™?
Yes ___   No ___

If Yes, which ones?
_____
_____
_____

What other book(s) on eating disorders have you purchased? _____
_____
_____

Was this book:
___ more helpful than other(s)
___ less helpful than other(s)

Do you think this book was worth its price?
Yes ___   No ___

Did this book cover all topics related to eating disorders adequately?
Yes ___   No ___

Please explain your answer:
_____
_____
_____

Were there any specific sections in this book that were of particular help to you?   Yes ___   No ___

Please explain your answer:
_____
_____
_____

On a scale of 1 to 10, with 10 being the best rating, how would you rate this guide? ___

What other titles would you like to see published in the _Unofficial Guide_™ series?
_____
_____

Are Unofficial Guides™ readily available in your area?   Yes ___   No ___

Other comments:
_____
_____
_____
_____

Get the inside scoop...with the *Unofficial Guides*™!

Health and Fitness

The Unofficial Guide to Alternative Medicine
ISBN: 0-02-862526-9 Price: $15.95

The Unofficial Guide to Conquering Impotence
ISBN: 0-02-862870-5 Price: $15.95

The Unofficial Guide to Coping with Menopause
ISBN: 0-02-862694-x Price: $15.95

The Unofficial Guide to Cosmetic Surgery
ISBN: 0-02-862522-6 Price: $15.95

The Unofficial Guide to Dieting Safely
ISBN: 0-02-862521-8 Price: $15.95

The Unofficial Guide to Having a Baby
ISBN: 0-02-862695-8 Price: $15.95

The Unofficial Guide to Living with Diabetes
ISBN: 0-02-862919-1 Price: $15.95

The Unofficial Guide to Overcoming Arthritis
ISBN: 0-02-862714-8 Price: $15.95

The Unofficial Guide to Overcoming Infertility
ISBN: 0-02-862916-7 Price: $15.95

Career Planning

The Unofficial Guide to Acing the Interview
ISBN: 0-02-862924-8 Price: $15.95

The Unofficial Guide to Earning What You Deserve
ISBN: 0-02-862523-4 Price: $15.95

The Unofficial Guide to Hiring and Firing People
ISBN: 0-02-862523-4 Price: $15.95

Business and Personal Finance

The Unofficial Guide to Investing
ISBN: 0-02-862458-0 Price: $15.95

The Unofficial Guide to Investing in Mutual Funds
ISBN: 0-02-862920-5 Price: $15.95

The Unofficial Guide to Managing Your Personal Finances
ISBN: 0-02-862921-3 Price: $15.95

The Unofficial Guide to Starting a Small Business
ISBN: 0-02-862525-0 Price: $15.95

Home and Automotive

The Unofficial Guide to Buying a Home
ISBN: 0-02-862461-0 Price: $15.95

The Unofficial Guide to Buying or Leasing a Car
ISBN: 0-02-862524-2 Price: $15.95

The Unofficial Guide to Hiring Contractors
ISBN: 0-02-862460-2 Price: $15.95

Family and Relationships

The Unofficial Guide to Childcare
ISBN: 0-02-862457-2 Price: $15.95

The Unofficial Guide to Dating Again
ISBN: 0-02-862454-8 Price: $15.95

The Unofficial Guide to Divorce
ISBN: 0-02-862455-6 Price: $15.95

The Unofficial Guide to Eldercare
ISBN: 0-02-862456-4 Price: $15.95

The Unofficial Guide to Planning Your Wedding
ISBN: 0-02-862459-9 Price: $15.95

Hobbies and Recreation

The Unofficial Guide to Finding Rare Antiques
ISBN: 0-02-862922-1 Price: $15.95

The Unofficial Guide to Casino Gambling
ISBN: 0-02-862917-5 Price: $15.95

All books in the *Unofficial Guide* series are available at your local bookseller, or by calling 1-800-428-5331.